How To Cut Children's Hair

Text and Illustrations

by

Larry Dunlap

IMPORTANT

PLEASE READ BEFORE

PROCEEDING

WITH ANY HAIRCUTTING:

<u>Terms of Use and Liability</u>

The information and techniques in this book are meant as a guide for responsible adults age 18 years or older to use on their own children.

It is not a substitute for the services of a professional, licensed cosmetologist.

No warranties or guarantees are made or implied regarding the results obtained by the purchaser or user, as a result of utilizing any of the information or techniques contained in "How To Cut Children's Hair".

Personal injury resulting from the use of information contained in this book, either to the person performing the haircut or the person receiving the haircut, are the sole responsibility of the purchaser or user.

Use of any of the information or techniques described in "How To Cut Children's Hair" constitutes acceptance of these terms and conditions. The author and/or any of his representatives accept no responsibility for any claims resulting from acceptance of these terms and conditions or use of the techniques in this book.

If these terms are not accepted, purchaser may return your hard copy of "How To Cut Children's Hair" to the place of purchase, prior to use and at their expense, for a full refund.

How to Use This Book

"How to Cut Children's Hair" was designed to teach the fundamental techniques needed to create virtually any type of haircut.

To get the best results begin by reading:

Chapter 1 "What You Will Need" to be certain that you have the necessary tools.

Chapter 2 "Controlling Your Child" which wil give you some handy tips on getting your child to co-operate during the cutting process.

Chapter 3 "The Basics" to get an overview of fundamentals like how to make straight parts, the correct way to hold the scissors and other essential skills.

Chapter 4 "Bangs" will teach you how to cut a basic bang shape. Most of the haircuts refer back to this chapter, so it's a good idea to read through it before proceeding.

Once you have read the first four chapters, decide which of the haircuts is closest to what you want to achieve by taking a look ct the illustrations at the beginning of each haircutting chapter. Be sure to take note of which version you are going to do and read the notes accompanying the illustration.

Read the entire chapter for the haircut you've chosen <u>before</u> you begin. Then bookmark any pages you will have to refer to while cutting.

Have fun!

For more information on children's haircutting, videos and deals on haircutting tools visit www.HowToCutChildrensHair.com

Table of Contents

Table of Contents

Foreword

Haircutting can be a lot of fun. After thirty-one years of hairdressing I still get a kick out of making a dramatic change in someone's appearance. The sense of satisfaction after creating a well crafted cut has not diminished for me after all these years.

These same techniques can be used just as effectively for adults as well as children, so don't be afraid to try them out on your grown up friends and family. Practice on the kids first though, they're a lot more forgiving of "the learning curve".

It is my hope that you will find my book easy to follow and useful for years to come.

Thanks to all who were involved in this project. Special thanks to: Leslie Dunlap (wife and general life manager), Butch Dunlap and Rene Kirkwood (my patient and talented reference photographers) , Joan Ipock (word processing and scribble deciphering), and Lynn McKnight (text editing). .Also, extra special thanks to my models: Chelsea Dunlap, Zachary Dunlap, Robert Patterson, Eric Patterson, Tristan Patterson and Chelsea Saunders. Now that you are teenagers or older you may finally be over the trauma of being forced to sit still for such a long time.

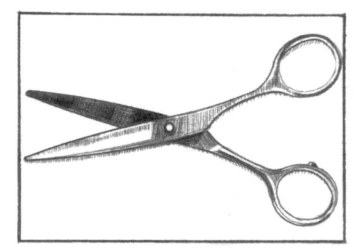

(Illustration 1): 5-inch Hair Cutting Scissors

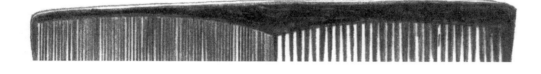

(Illustration 2): Hair Cutting Comb

What You Will Need

You can't make an omelet with a monkey wrench.

The proper tools can make any job a lot easier. Trying to give a haircut with your old household scissors is like trying to clean your driveway with a toothbrush. It can be done, but there must be an easier way.

The haircuts in this book can all be done with a few inexpensive tools. Make the investment now and you will be glad you did.

Following is a short list of things you will need. The first four items can be found at the local beauty salon equipment and supply store. You probably already have everything else you will need in your home.

Haircutting Scissors - Beauty salon supply stores always carry an inexpensive line of scissors designed for beauty school students. You can buy a perfectly good pair for under $25 that will work well through hundreds of haircuts. I recommend 5-inch long scissors, either with or without a pinkie rest (Illustration 1). These should be used only for cutting hair, so hide them from your kids. You remember what happened to the good sewing scissors you bought, don't you?

Combs - Look for a rigid, standard size, haircutting comb. Buy two or three in case you break one. If your child has dark hair, buy a light colored comb. If your child has light hair buy a dark colored comb. If you're cutting more than one child's hair and one is light, the other dark, buy a grey comb. The idea is to use a comb that is a contrasting color to your child's hair color. This makes it easier to see the ends of the hair while cutting.

Always use the wide spaced teeth when doing a haircut. This produces less tension on the hair and results in a more even cut.

Chapter 1 / What You Will Need

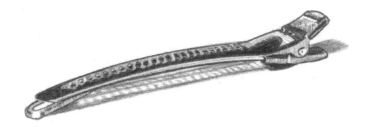

(Illustration 3): <u>Clips</u> - You will need six 4-inch alligator clips--four for the hair, two for the kids' toes (I'll explain later)

<u>Clips</u> - It's far easier to cut hair in small sections. Clips are necessary For all but the very shortest haircuts. You will need six four-inch alligator clips (Illustration 3). These work fine for most heads of hair, but long, thick hair is easier with butterfly clips. If you are planning on doing boys and girls cuts, get six of each.

<u>Haircutting Cape</u> - This makes your job easier by keeping the hair off your child's neck, resulting in less squirming, scratching, and whining, thus reducing your desire to choke them. Try to remember, choking your child is illegal, even if you just choke them a little bit.

<u>Water Sprayer</u> - You will need one for rewetting the hair as you work. anything that sprays water will do--even a water pistol. Come to think of it, especially a water pistol. You're dealing with kids remember?

<u>Chair</u> - Use any chair that will bring your child closest to your eye level. A bar stool works quite well. Very small children may need a person on that stool to hold them--a very patient person.

<u>Razor</u> - This refers to a razor (shaver) like you would shave a man's face with, <u>not</u> an electric razor or clippers. Whatever you have around the house will work. You will only need it for cleaning up the neck area of short haircuts.

<u>A Place to Work</u> - Select a work area that is well lit from all angles. Place the cutting stool in an area where you can move freely around it.

Make sure you work in front of a mirror. Looking at your child in the mirror is the easiest way to see if your cutting is balanced. Somehow it's easier to notice mistakes in the reflected image (Illustration 4).

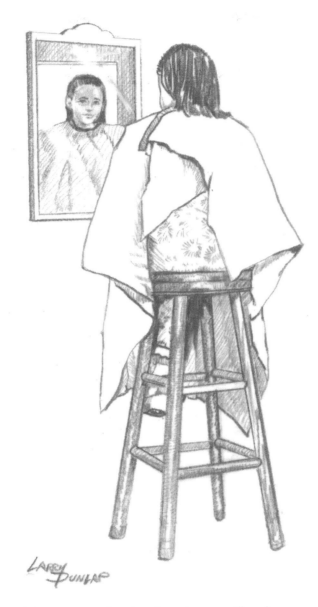

(Illustration 4): Preparing a functional work area will make
your job easier and more enjoyable.

Optional Tools

The following tools are not absolutely essential to achieve the haircuts in this book. All of the techniques described can be done with scissors and a comb. However, these additional tools can be helpful.

<u>Thinning Shears</u> - These are used at the end of a haircut to remove the bulk, provide soft texture or to create spiky looks without changing the overall length. See Chapter 10, "Finishing Touches" for additional information (page 136).

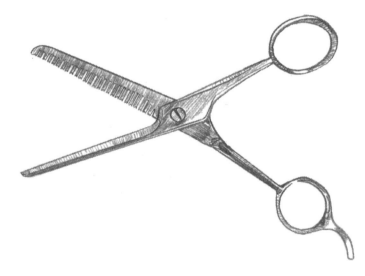

(Illustration 5): <u>Thinning Shears</u>.

Small Edging Clippers - These can be used to trim the ear and neckline areas of short haircuts. They also work well for shaving necks and sideburns.

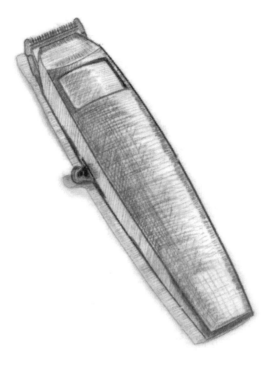

(Illustration 6): Small Edging Clippers .

<u>Large Tapering Clippers and Guide Attachments</u> - These can be used to create very short, military style haircuts or to quickly cut the shortest areas of a haircut. The clip-on guides determine the length of the area to be cut. They generally are numbered from one-five. A number one guide will cut the hair extremely short (almost bald); a number five will leave the hair about 1/2 inch to 3/4 inches long. Always cut against the growth direction.

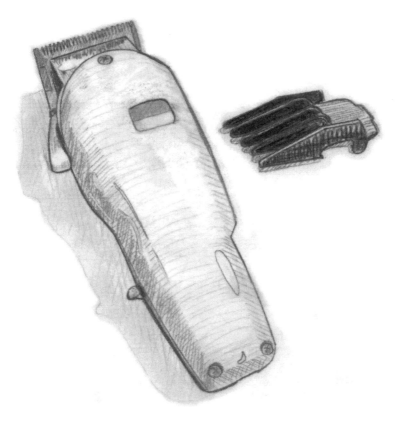

(Illustration 7): <u>Large Tapering Clippers and Guide</u> .

For more information on children's haircutting, videos and deals on haircutting tools visit
www.HowToCutChildrensHair.com

Chapter 2

Controlling Your Child

Haircuts sometimes bring out the worst in children. On occasion even the most good-natured child will squirm, twist, caterwaul, and hip-hop their way through the entire process. An uninformed observer might mistake your attempts at a bang trim for an exorcism.

Instead of ropes or prescription sedatives, try keeping in control with some of the following ideas:

The Bribe - A tried and true classic that almost always helps. Don't bribe with lollipops, they get all hairy and gross.

Busy Hands - Give your child something to hold for you, like your clips or the sprayer. The mirror is good for water pistol practice.

Positioning Your Child's Head - While working on the side areas, you will probably need your child's head tilted to the side.

Try gently pushing the head to the side and what happens? The whole body tilts sideways and they fall off the stool.

Here's the trick--with one hand firmly holding the shoulder, nudge your child's head over with your free hand. Remember this one because you will use it a lot.

Look Down Please - While working in the nape area, you will need the head tilted forward. It's not as simple as it sounds.

Try this. Reach around and pull the child's chin down with one hand while nudging the head forward with the other hand. Say, "Look down at the floor and don't move until I tell you to."

Toe Clips - If the above method doesn't work, take one of your extra clips, show it to the child to get his attention, then quickly reach down and clip it to his toes. When the kid bends down to remove the clip, attack that neckline like a person possessed. Repeat as necessary.

Hold the Ball for Me - This is a variation of the Toe Clips trick. Use a tennis ball or other similar sized ball. Say, "Can you hold this ball under your chin while I count to twenty?" Again, while their chin is down, cut like the wind!

The Safety Hold - Working around your child's eyes and ears can be dangerous if he is being wiggly. Use your free hand to firmly hold the top of his head while cutting in sensitive areas. With very small children, get the person holding them to do it for you (Illustration 8).

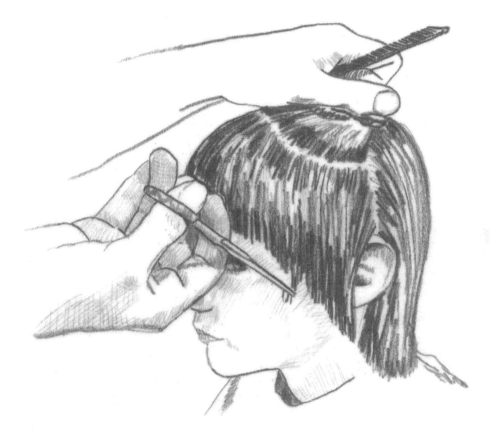

(Illustration 8): The Safety Hold

Know When to Quit - If your kid is throwing a tantrum or otherwise acting like your spouse's side of the family, call it quits. If you continue you'll be mad, the kid will be mad and he will have a rotten haircut to boot!

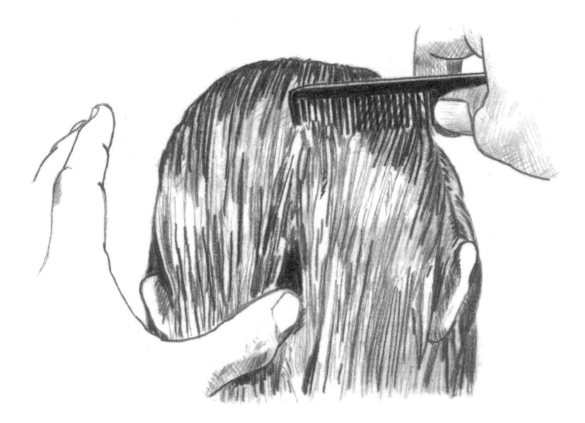

(Illustration 9): Place your thumb where you want the part to end and comb towards it.

Chapter 3

The Basics

Even a journey of a thousand miles must begin with the first snip.

All of the haircuts in this book, as varied in final appearance as they are, require the use of the same set of basic skills. Take time to review these basics so that you will be familiar with them when you are actually giving a haircut.

Most of the techniques are re-explained in other chapters to minimize page turning on your part.

Icons are included in some illustrations as an aid to remembering the basics. These are illustrated and explained later in this chapter.

Making Straight Partings

In order to easily create straight partings, place the tip of your comb where you want the part to begin. Place the thumb of your free hand where you want the part to end and pull the comb along the scalp until you touch your thumb (Illustration 9). Take some time to practice this now, I'll wait.

Sectioning

The main reason for sectioning during a haircut is to limit the amount of hair you are working with in order to give you more control of your work. This is the only time it is acceptable to be a control freak.

Most of the haircuts in this book begin with the same four basic sections.

First divide the hair in half by parting from behind one ear to the other across the top of the head.

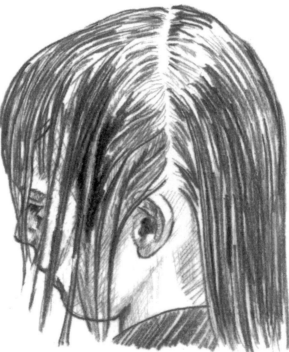

(Illustration 10): First divide the hair in half.

Next, subdivide the back by parting from center top to center neckline.

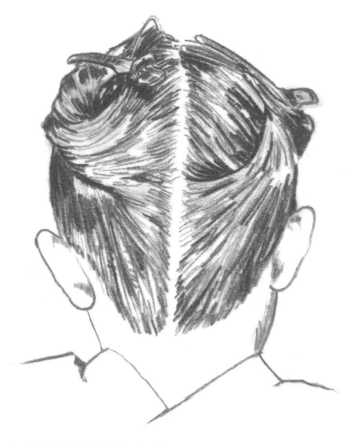

(Illustration 11): Subdivide the back.

Finally, subdivide the front area by parting from center top to the center of the front hairline.

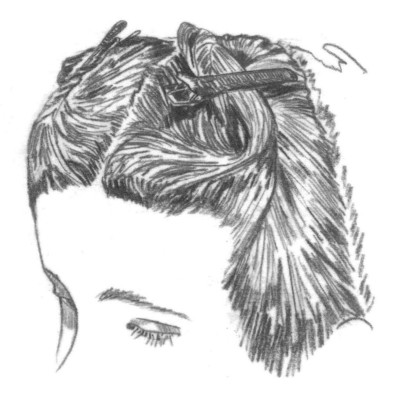

(Illustration 12): Subdivide the front area.

IMPORTANT: If the finished hairstyle is going to be worn with a definite part, use that part instead of a center part.

Holding the Hair

There are three basic ways to hold the hair while cutting:

Holding the Hair Against the Skin

The hair is simply combed flat against the skin and <u>if necessary</u>, held in place with one finger. The open scissors are slipped under the hair and the cut is made against the skin.

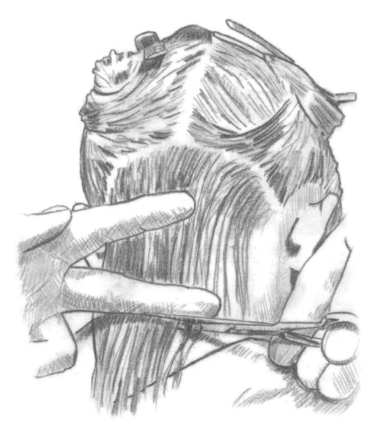

Illustration 13): Holding the hair against the skin.

Cutting on the Back of the Hand.

The hair is held between the middle and index fingers. The scissors are held parallel to the backs of the fingers for cutting.

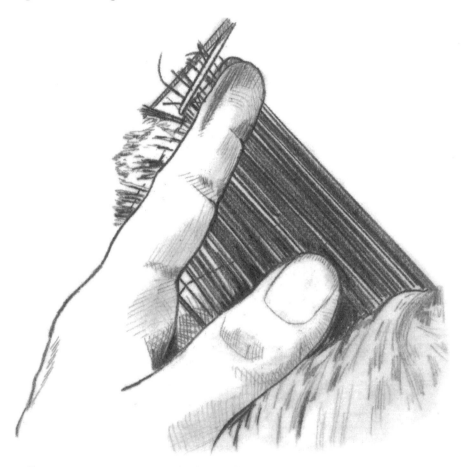

(Illustration 14): <u>Cutting on the back of the hand</u>.

Cutting Inside the Palm

The hair is held between the middle and index fingers. The scissors are held parallel to the insides of the fingers for cutting.

Unless specified for a particular haircut, cutting on the back of the hand or inside the palm is a matter of personal preference. Try each way to see which feels more natural to you.

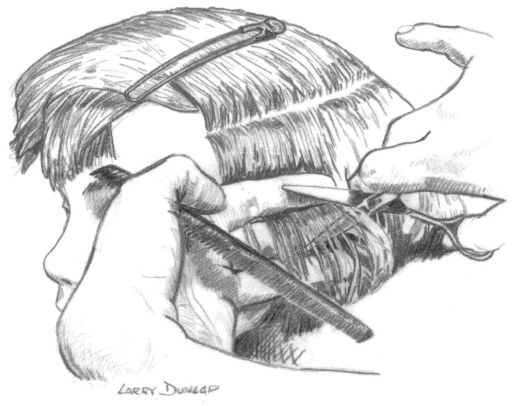

(Illustration 15): <u>Cutting inside the palm</u>.

IMPORTANT NOTE: When cutting hair held between your fingers, be sure to cut only in the area between your middle joint and finger tips.

You can't hold the hair tightly enough in the space next to the hand to achieve a precise cut. Observing this rule will also reduce the likelihood of cutting your hand (Illustration 16).

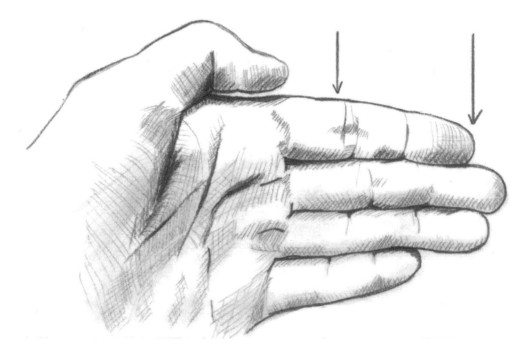

(Illustration 16): Cut only in the area between your middle joint

Cowlicks and Unruly Hair:
The Bend Test.

Many times while giving a haircut, you may have questions similar to these. "How much length can I remove without causing the hair to stick out? Can I cut the bangs short enough to stay out of the eyes but still have enough to style away from the face? How short does the hair have to be to spike? How do you control cowlicks?"

The answers to these and similar questions can be determined by this simple test of the hair's natural bend. Grasp a strand of hair from the area in question at a point about two inches from the scalp. Push the hair strand toward the scalp and observe where it bends (Illustration 17).

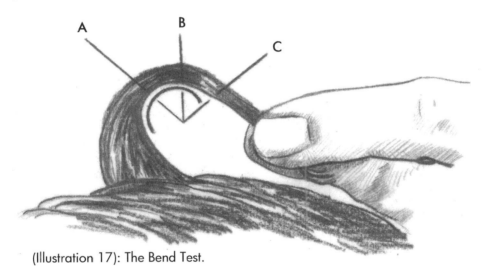

(Illustration 17): The Bend Test.

A. Cutting below the midpoint of the bend could cause the hair to spike or stick up.

B. Cutting ½ to ¾ inch beyond the midpoint of the bend leaves enough length for the hair to lie down.

C. Cutting 1 inch or more above the midpoint of the bend leaves enough length for the hair to lie down and be styled in a definite direction.

IMPORTANT NOTE: Hair texture is always an important consideration. Coarse, thick hair will require more length to lie smoothly than will fine, thin hair. If you are still in doubt after performing this test, try leaving a little extra length. You can always cut more later.

You will see the "Bend Test" icon at appropriate places in the illustrations as a reminder to use this useful way of determining length (Illustration 18).

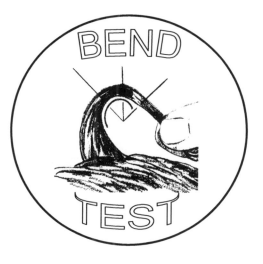

Illustration 18): <u>The Bend Test Icon</u>.

How to Hold Your Scissors

<u>How to Hold Your Scissors</u> - Very simply, your thumb and ring finger go in the holes. Use your index finger to steady the blades as you cut.

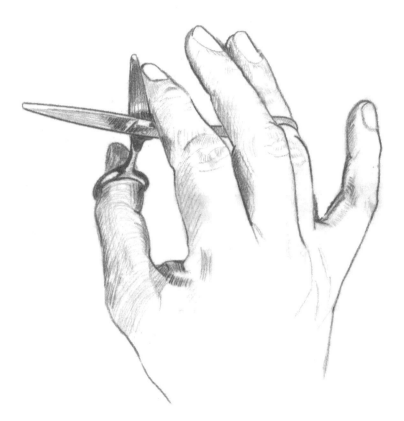

(Illustration 19): How to Hold Your Scissors

Scissors

<u>Blade Angle</u> - The angle of the scissor blade-surface in relation to how the hair is held is critical to the final result.

We have all seen women with bouncy shoulder-length hair that stays effortlessly turned under no matter what they're doing. Undercutting creates that style, and the blade angle is the key.

There are four basic blade angles:

<u>Blunt Angle</u>. The scissor blades are held parallel to the surface of the floor. This angle is used when cutting against the skin, trimming ends, etc. You will see the "Blunt Angle" icon at appropriate places in the illustrations as a reminder of the correct scissor angle to use.

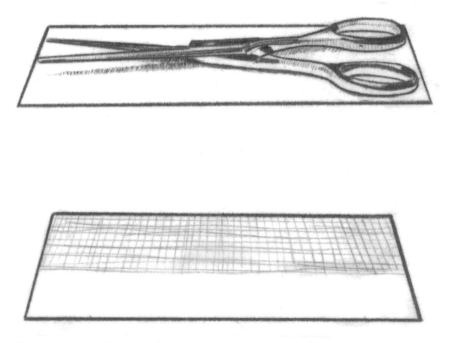

(Illustration 20): <u>Blunt Angle</u>.

Blade Angles

Undercut Angle. The scissor blades are held at a 45° angle so that the edge closest to your child's head is higher than the edge closest to you. This technique is used to create lines that turn under smoothly and easily. You will see the "Undercut Angle" icon at appropriate places in the illustrations as a reminder of the correct scissor angle to use.

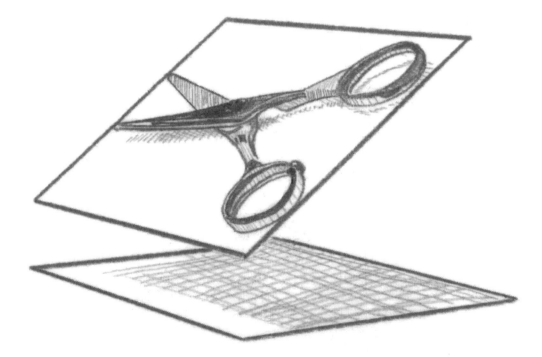

(Illustration 21): Undercut Angle.

Vertical Angle. The scissor blades are held at a right angle to the surface of the floor. This angle can be used to create dramatic wedge-type lines. You will see the "Vertical Angle" icon at appropriate places in the illustrations as a reminder of the correct scissor angle to use.

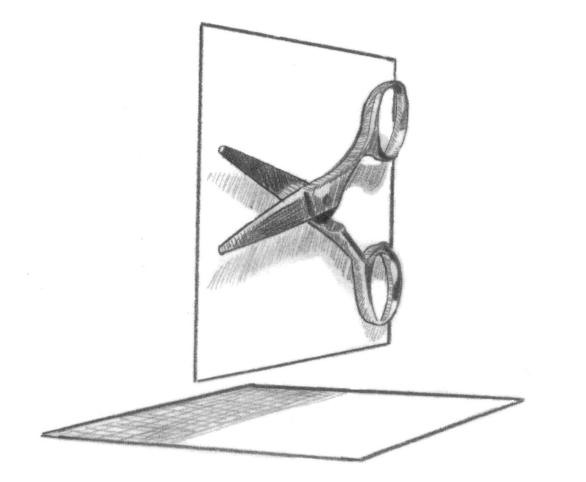

(Illustration 22): Vertical Angle.

<u>Diagonal</u>. The same as vertical but with the <u>length</u> of the scissors held at a diagonal. This is often used when layering short necklines. You will see the "Diagonal" icon at appropriate places in the illustrations as a reminder of the correct scissor angle tc use.

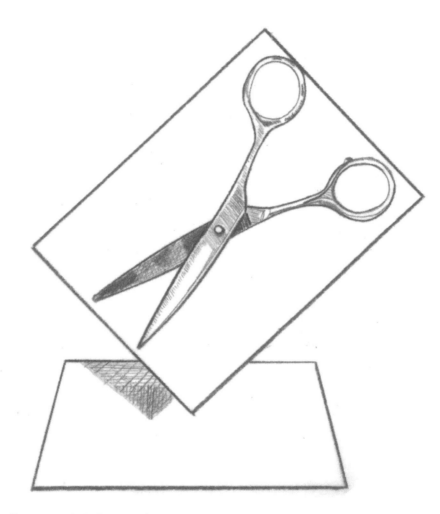

(Illustration 23): <u>Diagonal</u>.

Don't Stretch the Hair

The hair must be held with a minimal amount of tension while cutting. Lightly comb each section two or three times <u>with the wide spaced teeth</u> only (the fine teeth create too much tension) and then hold the hair without stretching it.

Learn to be conscious of this now, as holding the hair too tightly is a hard habit to break once you're used to it.

Overstretching the hair during cutting will cause the naturally elastic hair to snap back to its original shape and growth pattern, leaving behind an uneven or overly short cut. Particular care should be taken with naturally curly or wavy hair as it is especially elastic.

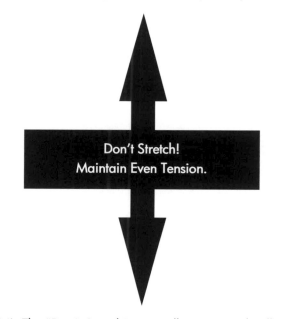

(Illustration 24): The "Don't Stretch" icon will appear in the illustrations occasionally as a reminder.

How to Check for Balance and Evenness

Often while cutting you may be unsure whether one side may be longer than the other. You may also have trouble deciding if a line is truly straight and even. When addressing these problems, there are two ways of looking at them:

First, there is visual balance and evenness. That is, upon visual observation the lines appear straight or the balance of length and weight appear the same from one side to another.

Secondly, there is technical balance and evenness. For example, if you measured the hair just behind each ear with a ruler, it might measure exactly 10 inches long from the scalp in both areas. This would be technically balanced and even.

Obviously, visual balance is of primary importance followed by the technical aspect. Sometimes when cutting you may be holding a section of hair that you have just cut and it appears perfectly even. However, when you release the hair and it returns to its natural growth direction, the line no longer "appears" even. Although the hair was technically correct, it was not visually even. With this in mind, two methods of checking for evenness and balance will be given: a visual method and a technical method. Rely mostly on the visual method and resort to the technical method when you are still in doubt.

Visual Checking

Position your child so that the area or areas in question are reflected in the mirror. Inspect the mirrored image for flaws rather than looking directly at your child's hair. When looking directly at something, you are seeing a three-dimensional image. When looking at a mirrored image, however, you are seeing a flattened, two-dimensional image. You will be surprised at how much easier it is to see flaws in this manner.

Technical Checking

To compare lengths from two areas that should be the same, try the following technique. Pick up a strand of hair from the same relative spot in each area between your thumb and index finger simultaneously.

Beginning next to the scalp, simultaneously slide both hands in unison down the hair shaft until your fingers slide off the tips of each strand (Illustration 25). If your fingers leave the ends at the same time, then the two strands are the same. If one hand leaves the ends before the other, then there is probably a difference in the lengths. Before making any corrections, check visually one more time.

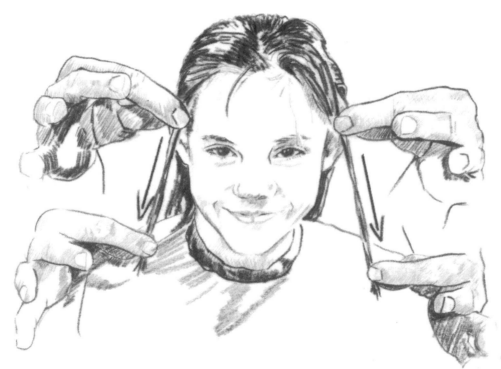

(Illustration 25): <u>Technical Checking</u>. Beginning next to the scalp, simultaneously slide both hands in unison down the hair shaft until your fingers slide off the tips of each strand.

For more information on children's haircutting, videos and deals on haircutting tools visit
www.HowToCutChildrensHair.com

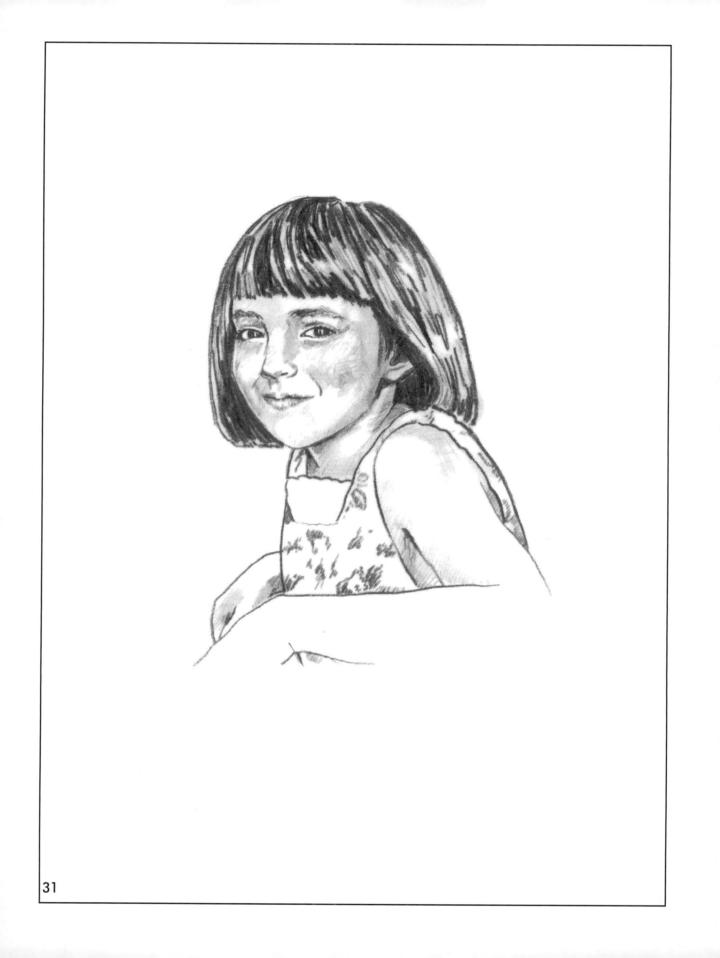

Bangs

If the eyes are like the windows looking into the soul, then the bangs must be the drapes.

The area of hair above the eyes is the most noticeable part of many haircuts and has a reputation for being difficult to cut.

Follow these simple steps and you will soon be trimming bangs like a pro.

Assemble all tools and prepare your work area. Your child's hair should be shampooed, conditioned and towel dried. Make sure the hair is damp but not wet.

Sectioning

Begin by parting off a triangular section above the eyes. To find the first point of your triangle, place your comb on top of the front of the head; center it above the nose (Illustration 26). Rock the comb back and forth and note where the comb touches the head while rocking. This is **Point A** of the triangle which denotes the highest point of the forehead. The hair tends to fall forward from this point into the eyes and should be included in the bangs.

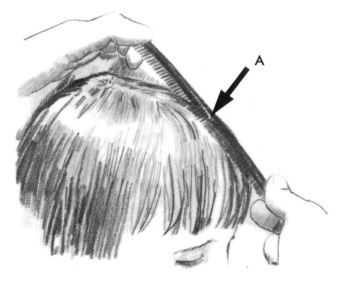

A

(Illustration 26): Finding the highest point on the forehead (Point A).

Now lift the hair on the forehead and find the two places on the hairline where the hair recedes. They are located above the outer corners of the eyes. Everyone has these, even kids. These places are **Points B and C** of your triangle.

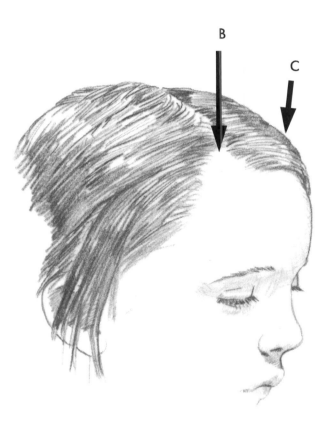

(Illustration 27): Find points B and C.

Part the hair from Point A to B and from Point A to C, creating a triangle.

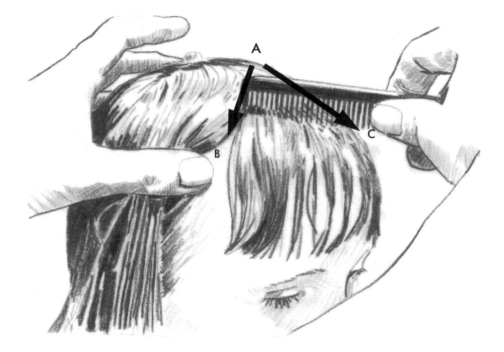

(Illustration 28): Create a triangular section.

Comb this hair down onto the forehead allowing it to lie in its natural growth pattern.

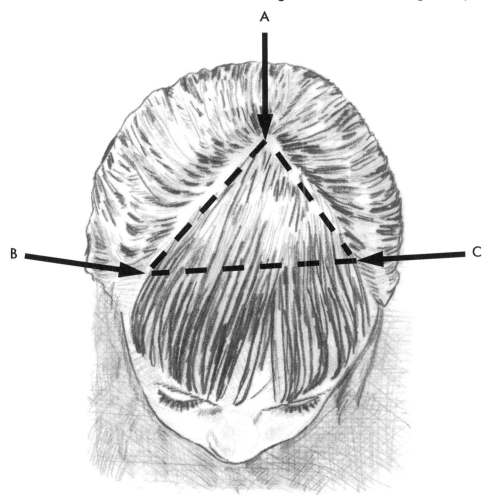

Illustration 29): Comb the hair straight down.

NOTE: Don't worry if the shape of your "triangle" isn't perfectly symmetrical. The human head is never perfectly balanced and your partings will reflect the natural asymmetries of your child's head.

Bang Length

Study the diagram to determine which length will best suit your child (Illustration 30).

     A. Bangs to be worn straight down on the forehead

     B. Bangs to be worn to the side or away from the face

     C. Wavy or curly hair

Always leave hair about ¼ inch longer than your desired length to allow for shrinkage as the hair dries. Allow ½ to 1 inch for wavy or curly hair. Remember you can always take more off but you can't put it back on.

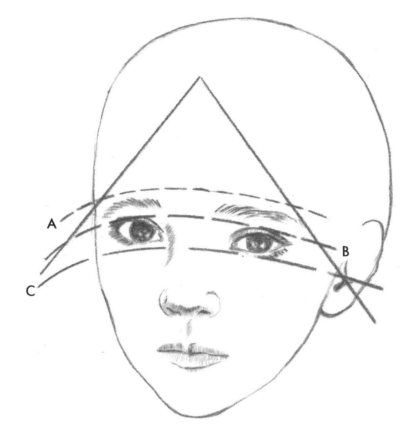

(Illustration 30): Choosing the right Bang Length

A. Bangs to be worn straight down on the forehead

B Bangs to be worn to the side or away from the face

C. Wavy or curly hair

IMPORTANT NOTE: Since you are using the eyebrows as a reference point for length, make certain your child's face is relaxed with the brows down (Illustration 31). If you cut while the eyebrows are in a "surprised" expression, the hair will be too short when the face is relaxed.

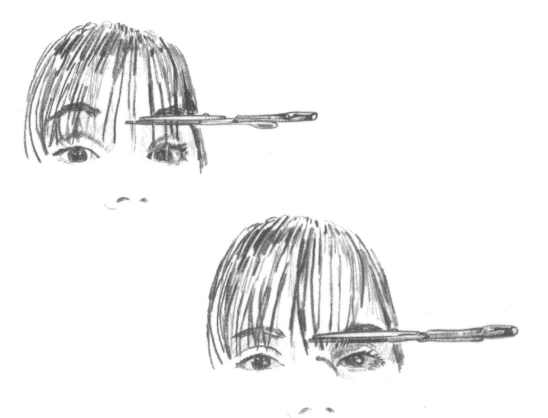

(Illustration 31): Make certain that the eyebrows (your guideline) are relaxed before cutting.

Cutting

Now you are ready to begin cutting. Use your comb and fingers to distribute the hair evenly across the forehead.

Place scissors at the outer corner of the eyes and begin cutting. Don't hold the hair in your hand; instead, use your free hand to steady your child's head while you cut. At this point you are trying to rough in the shape with the hair lying against the skin in its natural growth pattern in order to create a line that is *visually* even (Illustration 32).

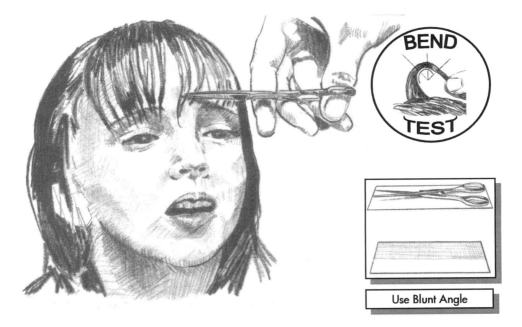

BEND TEST

Use Blunt Angle

(Illustration 32): Rough in the shape with the hair lying against the skin.

Once you are satisfied with the general shape of the bang, return to the outer corner of the eye. Lightly comb the previously cut hair and *without stretching* it, hold the hair between your fingers. Cut off any missed hairs without altering the established shape (Illustration 33).

If the bang appears crooked while you are holding it, release the hair, fluff it a little, and step back to take a look. If it appears straight, don't make any changes.

The basic bang is now complete. However, for lighter, more feathery bangs that can be styled away froe face you'll need to create some layers.

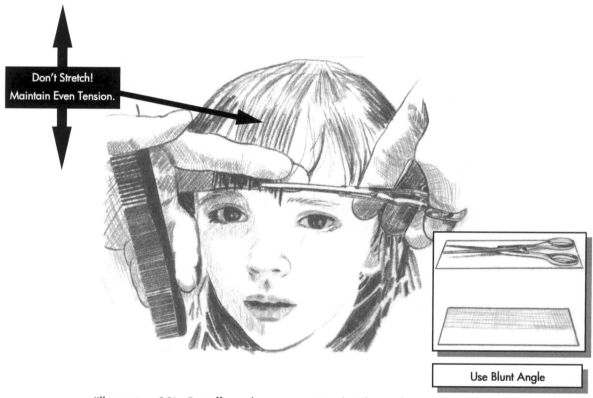

Don't Stretch!
Maintain Even Tension.

Use Blunt Angle

(Illustration 33): Cut off any hairs you missed without altering the established shape.

Pick up a ½-inch section of hair from the top of the triangle (Point A) to the center of the forehead and hold up and away from the head at a 90° angle (Illustration 34).

Layering the Bangs

Using the previously cut hair as your length guide, cut a line parallel to the surface of the head. *CONTINUE HOLDING THE HAIR.*

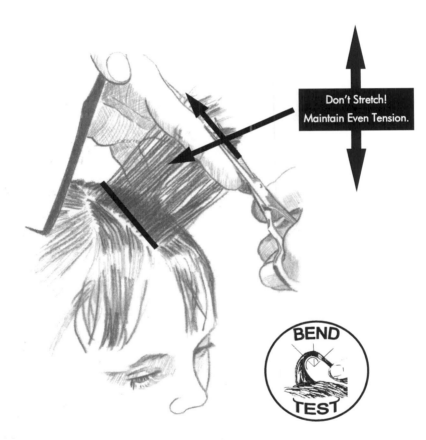

(Illustration 34): Cut a line parallel to the surface of the head.

Chapter 4 / Bangs

Combine hair from right of triangle with center hair and cut to match. Repeat with remaining hair on left of triangle and your bangs are completed!

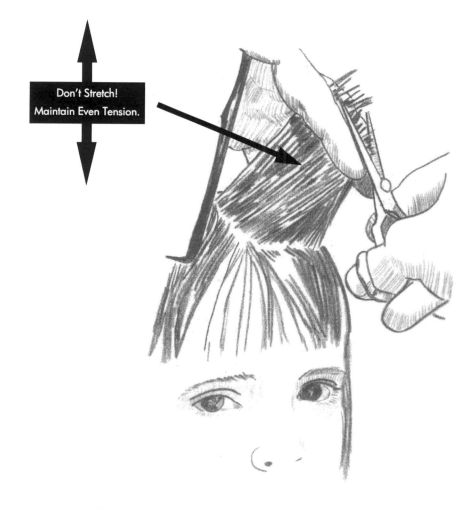

(Illustration 35): Cut the hair to match the center guideline.

Notes

For more information on children's haircutting, videos and deals on haircutting tools visit
www.HowToCutChildrensHair.com

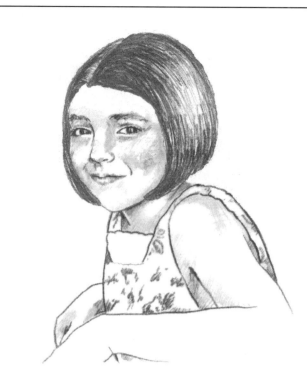

Use length option "A" for this hairstyle.

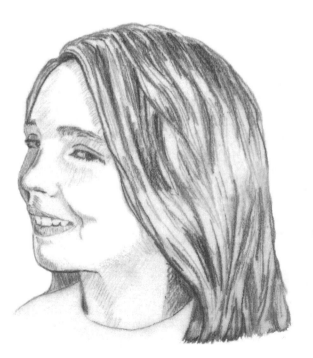

Use length option "B" for this hairstyle.

45

The Blunt Cut

The blunt cut is the simplest and most universal of all haircuts. Healthy, one-length hair will always look terrific and with a minimum of fuss.

If bangs are desired with the blunt cut, complete them first, following the directions in Chapter 4 (page 31).

Section clean, damp hair into the basic four sections (Chapter 3, page 13).

Sub-sections

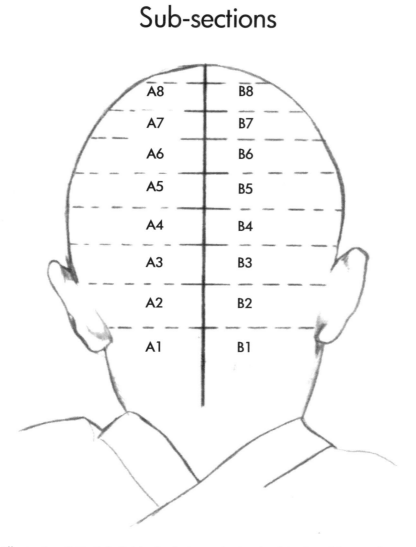

(Illustration 36): Subdivide the hair on the back of the head by combing sub-sections A1 and B1 down onto the neckline, leaving the remaining hair clipped up and away.

Mid-Shoulder Blade or Longer

If the desired finished length is mid-shoulder blade or <u>longer</u>, have your child <u>stand</u> with both feet flat and with both hands resting on a chair back or table top. This position enables your child to stand straight and steady while you cut (Illustration 37).

<u>IMPORTANT</u>: If the desired finished length is mid-shoulder blade or <u>shorter</u>, there is no need to have your child stand up for the haircut. Instead, have your child sit with her head bent slightly forward while you cut the back sections.

You may find it easier to kneel or sit while cutting in order to be at eye level while you work.

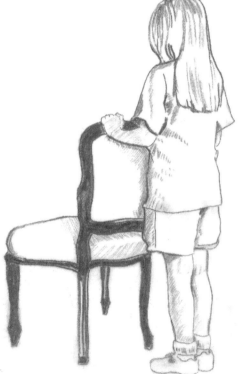

Illustration 37): If your child's hair is longer than mid-shoulder, have them stand while you cut.

Cutting the Back

Comb the hair from sub-sections A1 and B1 lightly to detangle and to align the hair strands. Hold the hair at the center of the sub-section between your index and middle fingers.

IMPORTANT: Throughout the cut make sure that you remember these two things.

1. Hold the hair firmly in a straight line but <u>without stretching</u>. Too much stretching will result in an uneven cut.

2. Make certain that the fingers holding the hair are resting firmly against the child's body while you are cutting. Resist the urge to hold the hair out and away from the body while cutting as this will result in an uneven haircut.

Now cut the hair to the desired length on a straight, horizontal line (Illustration 38).

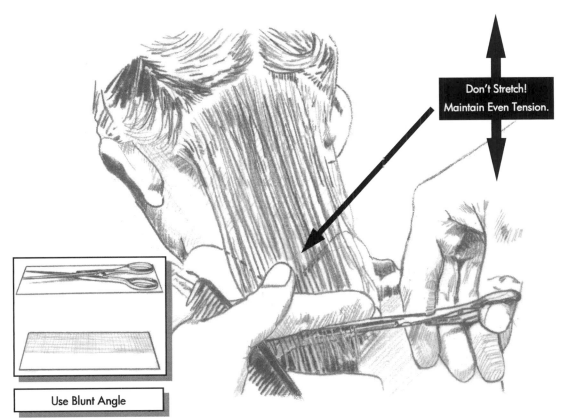

Don't Stretch!
Maintain Even Tension.

Use Blunt Angle

(Illustration 38): Cut to the desired length on a straight, horizontal line.

Chapter 5 / The Blunt Cut

When you complete your first sub-section (guideline), release the hair, have your child hold her head upright, then check for visual/technical evenness and straightness (Chapter 3, page 29). Remember that the length will appear about ½ inch shorter after the hair dries. Wavy or curly hair will shrink even more.

Make any necessary adjustments before proceeding. Next, drop down sub-sections C1 and D1 (Illustration 39). Make sure the sub-section is thin enough to allow you to see through to the previously cut hair (your guideline).

Combine the hair together and cut to match the guideline. Remember, no stretching, and keep the hair close to the body.

Continue sub-sectioning and cutting until the back sections are completed.

Cutting the Sides

(Illustration 39): Now subdivide sections C1 and D1.

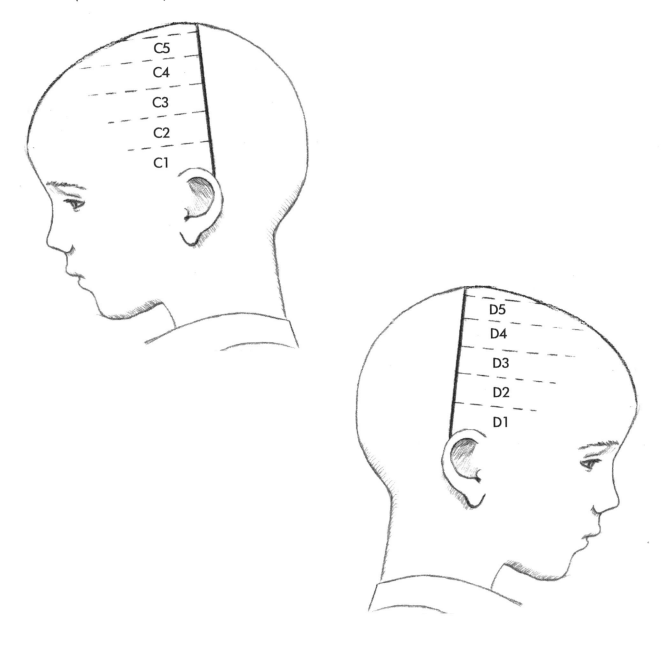

Chapter 5 / The Blunt Cut

With your child's head upright and tilted slightly away from you, comb the hair from sub-section C1 down and back so that it combines with the previously cut back section.

Using the previously cut hair in the back as your guideline, hold the hair between your fingers and cut on a horizontal line to match the back (Illustration 40). Remember not to stretch the hair.

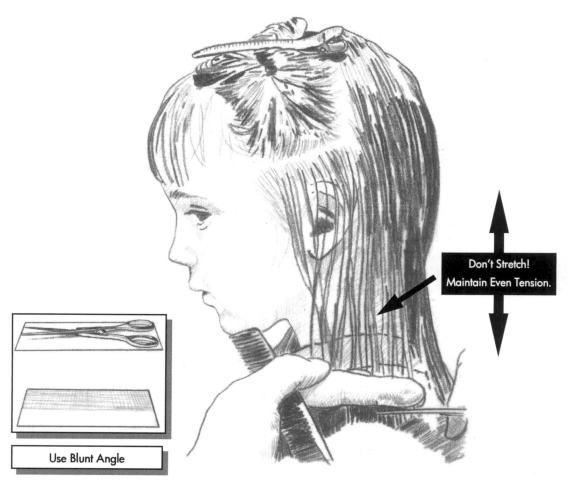

Use Blunt Angle

Don't Stretch!
Maintain Even Tension.

(Illustration 40): Hold the hair between your fingers and cut on a horizontal line to match the back.

Move to sub-section D1 and cut to match.

Now compare sub-sections C1 and D1 to see if lengths are visually and technically balanced (Chapter 3).

Next, drop down sub-sections C 2 and D2 and cut to match the previously cut hair (Illustrations 39 and 40).

Continue sub-sectioning and cutting in this manner until all the hair is evenly cut.

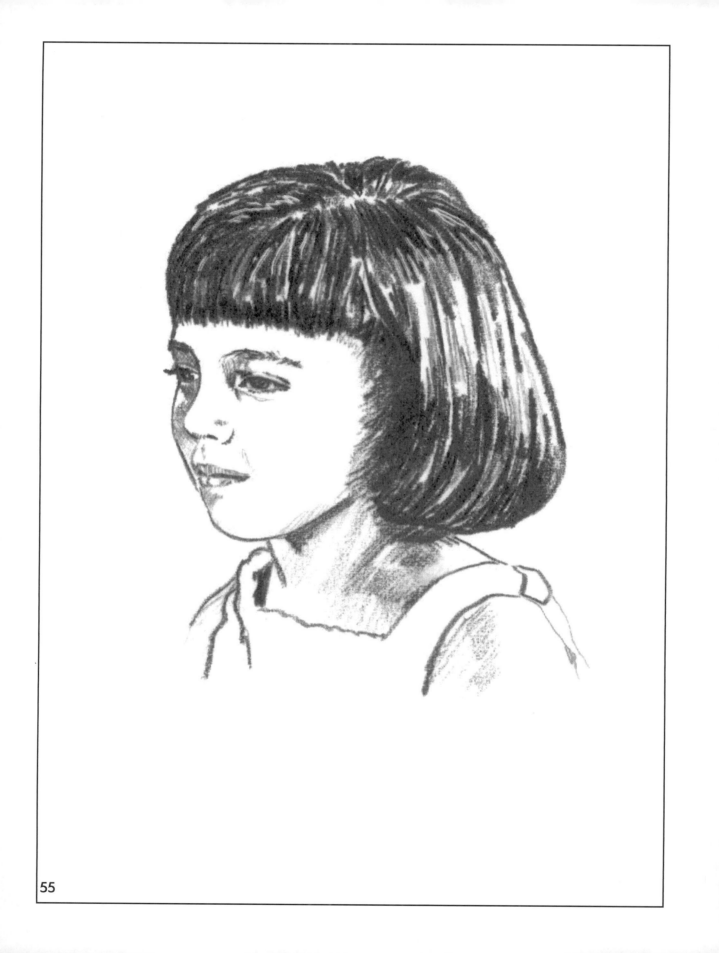

The Undercut

The undercut is a classic, easy-to-care-for hairstyle. Sometimes referred to as the "bob" or "page boy", it will create a full, turned under look that will always be in fashion.

The term "undercutting" refers to a method of haircutting that creates overlapping sections of hair that get progressively longer from the nape sections to the crown sections. This overlapping effect causes the hair to turn under more readily.

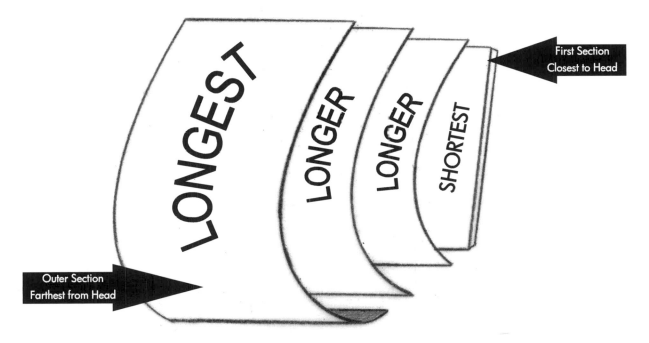

(Illustration 41): Undercutting

Determining the Length

When considering choosing this hairstyle, keep in mind that it is most effective on hair that is mid- shoulder length or shorter. Cutting the hair above the shoulder will create the most fullness.

Undercutting will not have a noticeable effect on <u>overly curly</u> hair. Blunt cutting is easier and more appropriate for very curly hair textures.

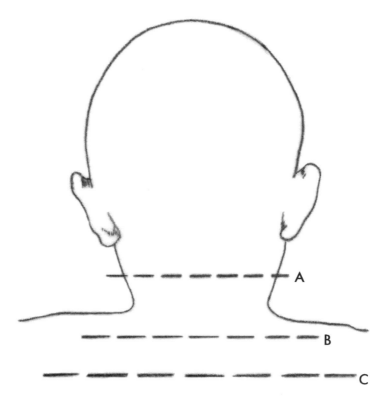

(Illustration 42): Study the diagram to determine which length will best suit your child.

    A. Provides maximum fullness, but is too short to be worn in a pony tail . Great for creating fullness in fine hair.

    B. Gives a smooth under turn, as well as a more versatile length. Good results for medium to thick hair. Less effective for fine hair.

    C. Will turn under with the aid of blow drying or curling. Long enough to easily stay behind shoulders and away from face.

Sub-Sections

If bangs are desired with the undercut, complete them first, following the directions in Chapter 4 (page 31).

To begin, assemble all tools and prepare your work area. Your child's hair should be shampooed, conditioned, and towel dried. Make sure the hair is damp but not wet.

Divide the hair into the four basic sections (Chapter 3, page 13).

Subdivide the hair on the back of the head by combing sub-sections A1 and B1 down onto the neckline, leaving the remaining hair clipped up and out of the way.

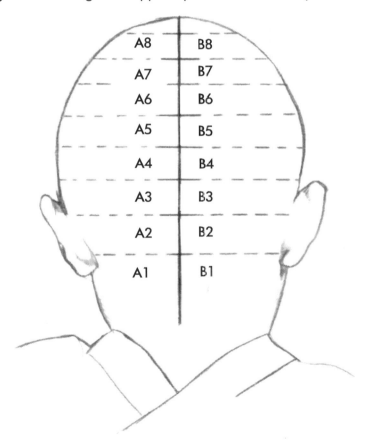

(Illustration 43): Subdivide the hair .

Cutting the Back

Comb the hair lightly to detangle and align the hair strands.

Allow the hair to lie against the skin in its natural growth pattern while cutting the first sections.

Without holding the hair, use the blunt scissor angle to cut the first section against the skin to the desired length. Your first section should be a horizontal line that is about ¾ inch shorter than the desired final overall length.

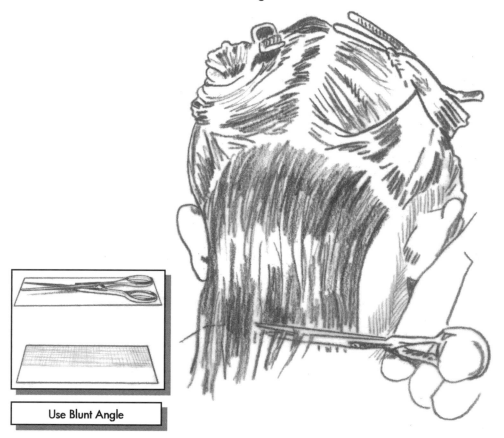

Use Blunt Angle

(Illustration 44): Your first section should be a horizontal line that is about ¾ inch shorter than the desired final overall length.

Check for visual evenness and balance (Chapter 3, page 29).

Now comb the previously cut hair smooth, hold it against the skin, and even out any missed hairs. Be sure not to make any major changes in the shape of the established line.

You now have an even guideline for the back.

Next, drop down sub-sections C1 and D1 (Illustration 43). Make sure this sub-section is thin enough to allow you to see through to your guideline underneath.

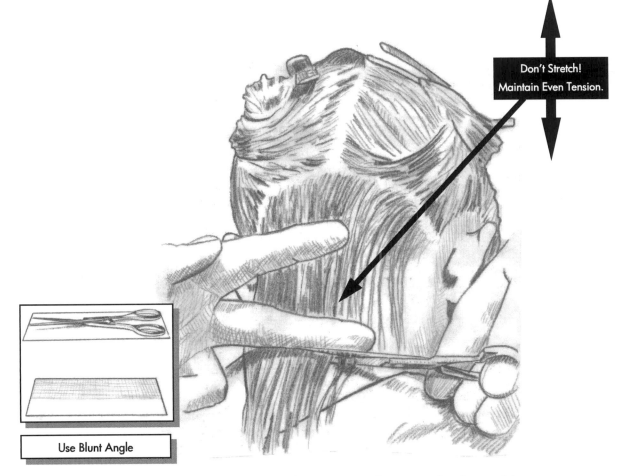

Don't Stretch!
Maintain Even Tension.

Use Blunt Angle

(Illustration 45): Be sure not to make any major changes in the shape of the established line.

Comb the hair together with the previously cut section. Hold the hair as shown.

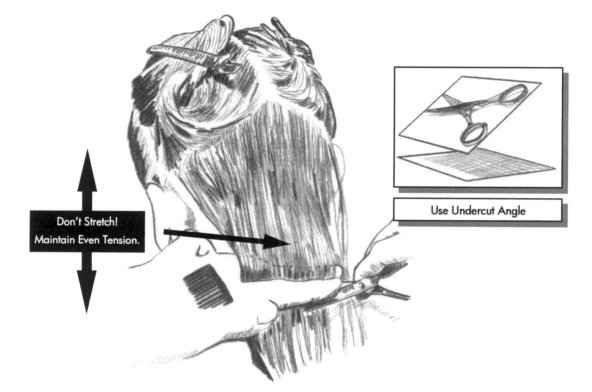

Don't Stretch!
Maintain Even Tension.

Use Undercut Angle

(Illustration 46): Comb the hair together with the previously cut section.
Hold the hair as shown.

Using the underscut scissor angle (page 24), cut this hair about ¼ inch longer than your guideline.

IMPORTANT:

1. Hold the hair in a straight line but without stretching. Too much stretching will result in an uneven cut.

2. Make certain that the fingers holding the hair are resting firmly against the child's body while you are cutting. Resist the urge to hold the hair out and away from the body while cutting as this will result in an uneven haircut.

Cutting the Sides

Check for visual and technical evenness and balance (Chapter 3, page 29).

Now drop down sub-sections 1E anD1F (Illustration 43).

Using the <u>undercut scissor angle</u> (page 24), cut to match the previously cut hair. Continue sub-sectioning and cutting until the back sections are completed.

Check for evenness and balance, making any necessary adjustments before proceeding to the side areas.

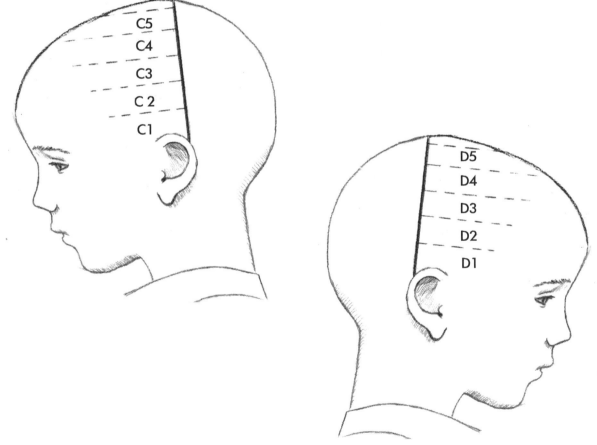

(Illustration 47): Now subdivide sections C1 and D1.

With your child's head upright and tilted slightly away from you, comb the hair from sub-section C1 down and back so that it combines with the previously cut back section.

Using the previously cut hair in the back as your guideline, hold the hair between your fingers and cut on a horizontal line to match the back (Illustration 48). Remember not to stretch the hair.

Now move to sub-section D1 and cut to match.

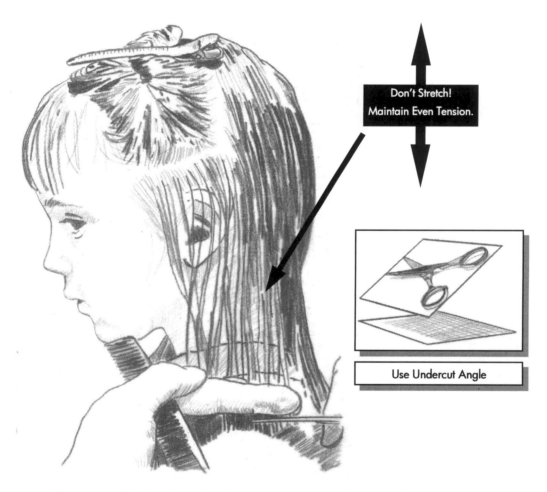

Don't Stretch!
Maintain Even Tension.

Use Undercut Angle

(Illustration 48): Comb the hair from sub-section C1 down and back so that it combines with the previously cut back section.

Now compare sub-sections C1 and D1 to see if lengths are visually and technically balanced (Chapter 3, page 29).

Next, drop down sub-sections C2 and D2 and cut to match the previously cut hair. Remember to use the <u>undercut scissor angle</u>.

Continue sub-sectioning and cutting in this manner until all of the hair is evenly cut.

Sub-sections

Now section clean, damp hair into the basic four sections (Chapter 3, page 13).

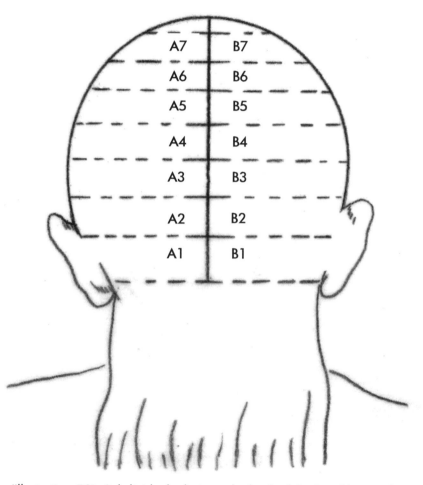

(Illustration 50): Subdivide the hair on the back of the head by combing sub-sections A1 and B1 down onto the neckline, leaving the remaining hair clipped up and out of the way.

Cutting the Back

Now, using the blunt scissor angle (Chapter 3, page 24), cut the hair to the desired length on a straight, horizontal line.

Comb the hair from sub-sections A1 and B1 lightly to detangle and to align the hair strands.

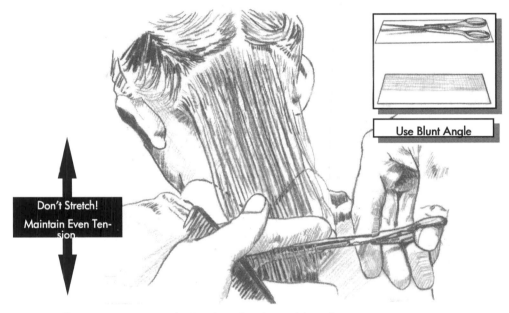

Don't Stretch! Maintain Even Tension

Use Blunt Angle

(Illustration 51): Cut the back to the desired length.

Hold the hair at the center of the sub-section.

- Hair that will be cut to the top of the shoulders or shorter should be cut against the skin while loosely held in place with one finger (page 16).

- Hair that will be cut shoulder length or longer should be held between your index and middle fingers (page 19).

<u>IMPORTANT</u>: While cutting the back sections, make sure you remember these two things.

1. Hold the hair firmly in a straight line <u>without</u> stretching.

2. Make certain that the fingers holding the hair are resting firmly against the child's body while you are cutting. Resist the urge to hold the hair out and away from the body while cutting as this will result in an uneven haircut.

Chapter 7 / The Angle Cut

When you complete your first sub-section (guideline), release the hair, have your child hold his/her head upright, then check for visual/technical evenness and straightness (page 29). Remember that the length will appear about ½ inch shorter after the hair dries. Wavy or curly hair will shrink even more.

Make any necessary adjustments before proceeding. Next, drop down sub-sections A2 and B2 (Illustration 50, page 67). Make sure the sub-section is thin enough to allow you to see through to the previously cut hair (your guideline).

Combine the hair together and cut to match the guideline. Remember, no stretching, and keep the hair close to the body.

Continue sub-sectioning and cutting until the back sections are completed.

Cutting the Front and Sides

Now subdivide sections C1 and D1.

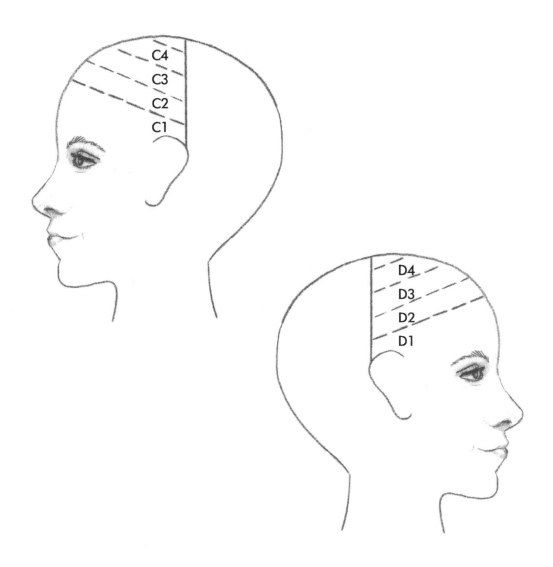

Chapter 7 / The Angle Cut

Stand in front of your child. Comb the hair from sub-section C1 toward your child's face. You are about to join your previously cut bang and back sections by cutting the sides on a diagonal line that blends the two areas (Illustration 53). The bang and back areas serve as your two guidelines.

IMPORTANT:

1. Hold the hair in a straight line but without stretching. Too much stretching will result in an uneven cut.

2. Make certain that the fingers holding the hair stay as close to the child's face as possible while cutting. Resist the urge to hold the hair out and away from the body while cutting as this will result in an uneven cut.

3. When blending the sides with the bang area, make certain that you are not removing hair from the bang area by cutting into it.

Hold the hair inside your palm and cut on the diagonal to join the previously cut guidelines.

Repeat with sub-section D1.

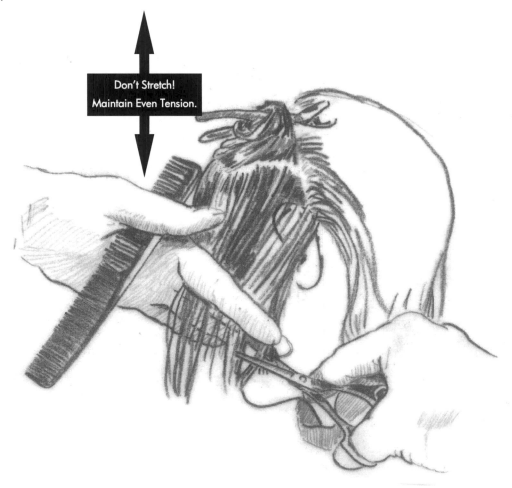

Don't Stretch!
Maintain Even Tension.

(Illustration 53): Cut on the diagonal to join the previously cut guidelines.

When you have completed sub-sections C1 and D1, comb the hair around the face downward allowing it to fall into its natural fall. Trim any pieces of hair that <u>drastically</u> deviate from the diagonal line. Small variations will disappear when the hair is dry.

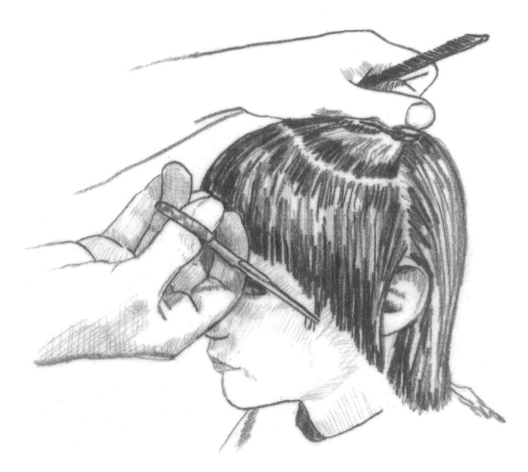

(Illustration 54): Trim any pieces of hair that <u>drastically</u> deviate from the diagonal line.

Next, check for visual and technical evenness and balance (Chapter 3, page 29).

Now drop down sub-sections C 2 and D2. Make sure these sub-sections are thin enough to allow you to see through to your guideline underneath.

Cut both sections to match your guidelines.

Continue sub-sectioning and cutting in this manner until the front sections are completed.

The <u>Basic Angled Cut</u> is now complete. To create more fullness and a softer look, continue with the Optional Layered Back (page 75).

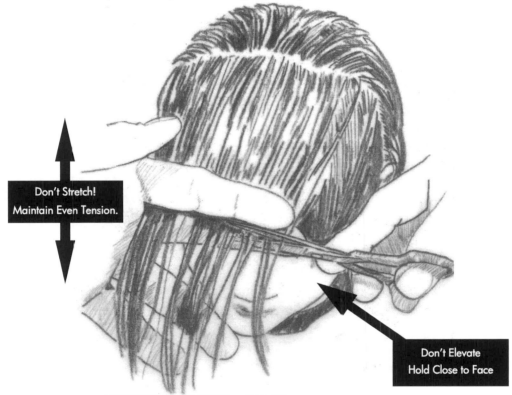

(Illustration 55): Comb the hair from <u>both</u> sub-sections forward so that it will overlap the bang section as well as the sides.

Optional Layered Back

The <u>Basic Angled Cut</u> leaves the back area with heavier, one-length hair. You may wish to soften and round out this area.

To begin, make sure the hair is still damp.

Stand in front of your child. Comb all of the hair from the back sections forward, over the top of the head. If the hair in the back is too thick to see through to your guideline, sub-section it for manageability.

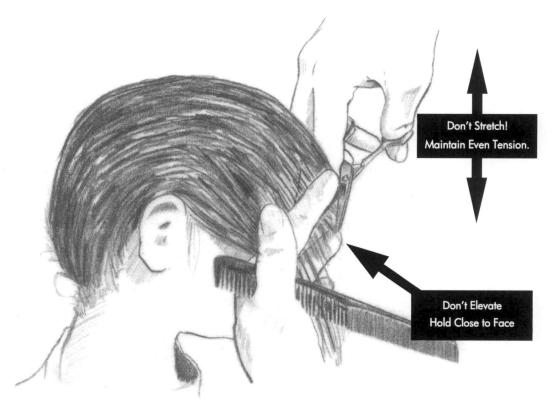

Don't Stretch!
Maintain Even Tension.

Don't Elevate
Hold Close to Face

(Illustration 56): Cut the hair from the back to match your guideline around the face.

If you desire a fuller, more rounded top area, continue with the <u>Optional Layered Top</u>.

Optional Layered Top

For hair that will be curled during styling, or for curly, wavy hair, the layered top will create a fuller, more rounded effect. This version of the angled haircut allows the most versatility in styling.

To begin, make sure the hair is still damp.

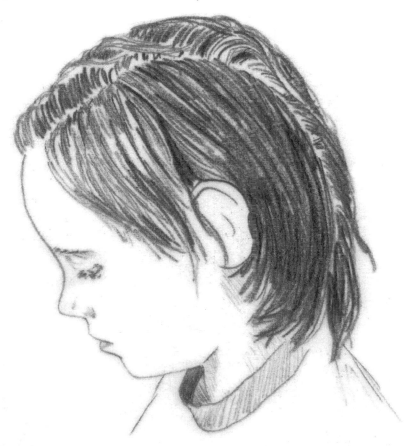

(Illustration 57): Create a "Mohawk" section about 1 inch wide along an imaginary line running from the center of the face to the middle of the back neckline.

Comb all other hair down and away from this section.

Stand at your child's side. Comb the hair straight up in the "Mohawk" area starting about 2 inches behind the front hairline to about 2 inches behind the crown area and grasp it between your fingers.

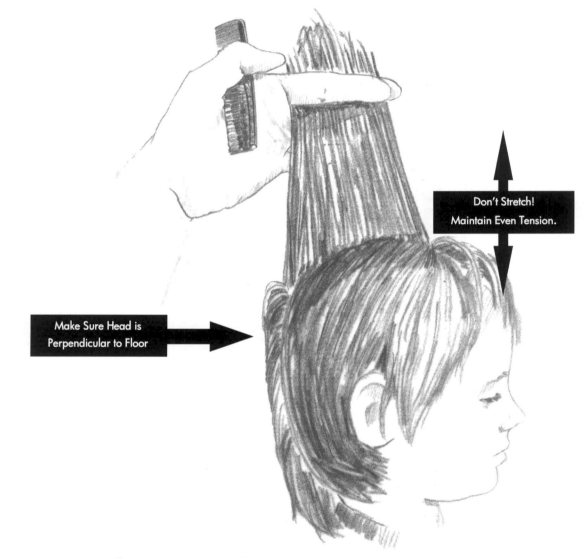

Don't Stretch!
Maintain Even Tension.

Make Sure Head is
Perpendicular to Floor

(Illustration 58): Comb the hair straight up.

Cut a line joining the shortest areas in this section. Make sure that your child's head is upright and straight, and that you are holding the hair in the center of the head along the "Mohawk" line.

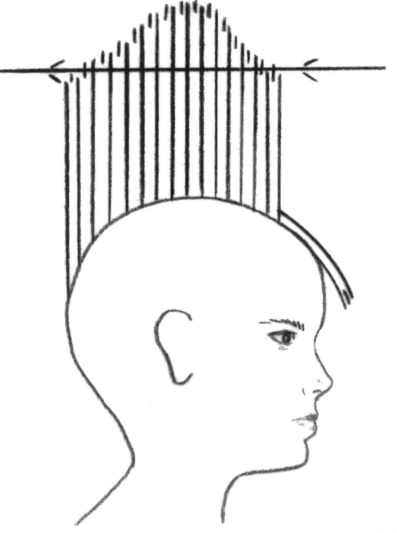

(Illustration 59): Cut a line joining the shortest areas in this section.

When the center guide is complete, stand behind your child and comb all of the hair straight back and away from the face.

Now combine hair from the hairline with the hair about 1 inch behind it and cut to match. You now have two guidelines to
follow: the center guideline and the previously cut hair from the front hairline.

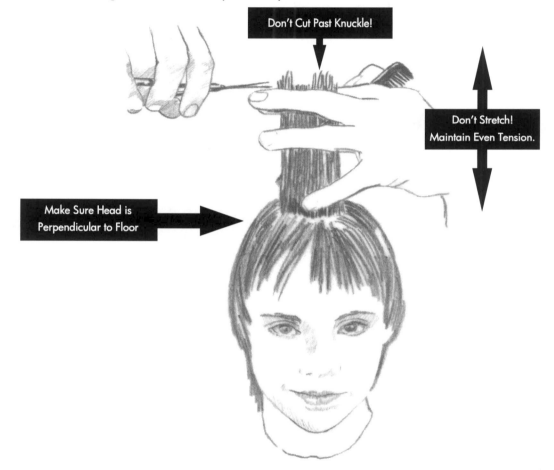

(Illustration 60): Combine hair from the hairline with the hair about 1 inch behind it and cut to match.

Now combine this previously cut hair with hair from about 1 inch behind it and cut to match. You now have two guidelines to follow--the center guideline and the previously cut hair from 1 inch behind the front hairline.

Continue cutting in this manner, moving toward the crown in 1-inch wedges until the top is completely blended.

For more information on children's haircutting, videos and deals on haircutting tools visit
www.HowToCutChildrensHair.com

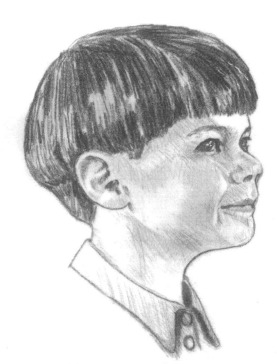

Use option "A" for shortest boy's version of the wedge.

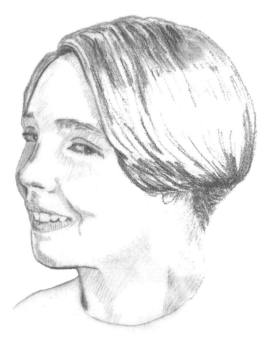

Use option "C" for this girls version of the wedge.
Optional top layering will create a softer haircut.

The Wedge

Also known as "The Bowl Cut", "Surfer Cut", and "Mushroom Cut", the wedge is a classic, easy-care haircut for girls and boys. The un-layered version of this cut is perfect for controlling unruly cowlicks.

Begin by cutting the bangs (Chapter 4, page 31).

When the bangs are completed, divide hair into the basic four sections (Chapter 3, Page 13), then subdivide section on right side of head as shown. If hair is long or excessively thick, make your sub-sections thinner.

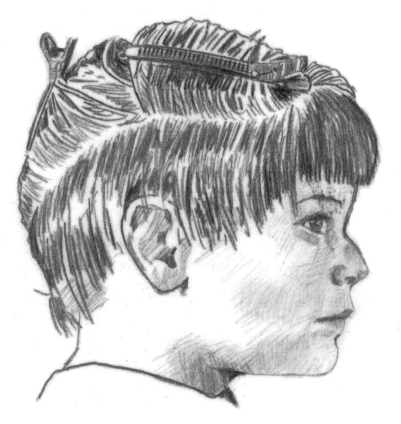

(Illustration 61): Divide hair into the basic four sections (Chapter 3, Page 13), then subdivide section on right side of head as shown.

Chapter 8 / The Wedge

The most important part of a wedge is the interior weight line. That's the fullest part of the finished cut that sort of "mushrooms out" above the close fitting neckline.

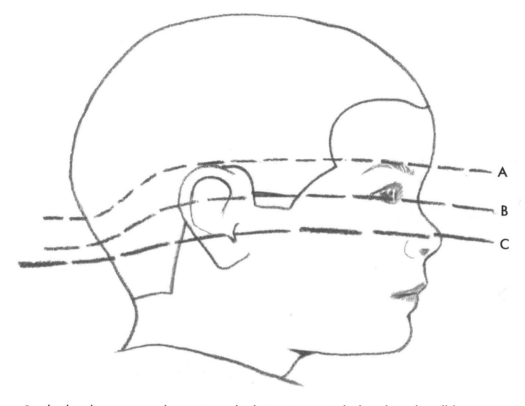

Study the diagram to determine which interior weight line length will best suit your child. All lengths can be worn turned under or styled away from the face.

    A. Shortest. The classic Wedge.

    B. Mid-length. Appropriate for boys or girls.

    C. Longest. Usually worn by girls. Offers more styling options.

This length won't determine the length on the neck. We'll worry about that later.

If you desire more length than is shown in Option C, the Angle Cut (Chapter 7, page 65) or Undercut (Chapter 6, page 55) are better choices.

Cutting the Interior Weight-Line

Begin at the ear by first combing up from underneath.

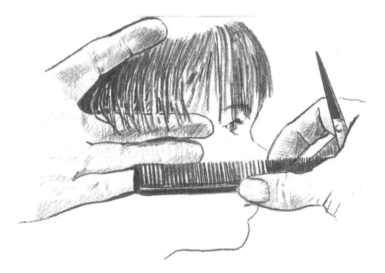

Then comb down from above.

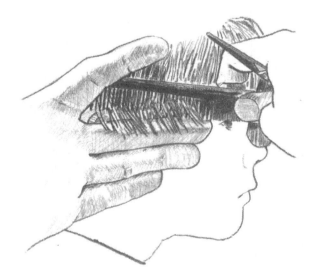

Grasp the hair between your fingers at the level of the desired length.

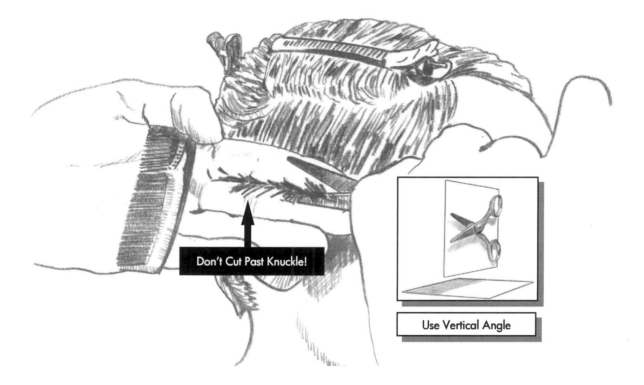

Don't Cut Past Knuckle!

Use Vertical Angle

(Illustration 65): Grasp the hair at the level of the desired length.

Now cut on a horizontal line from the temple to the back of the ear.

IMPORTANT: Make sure that the hand holding the hair is resting firmly against the child's head while cutting the weight line.

Next, move to just behind the ear and repeat this procedure. Remember to angle the line slightly downward at this point.

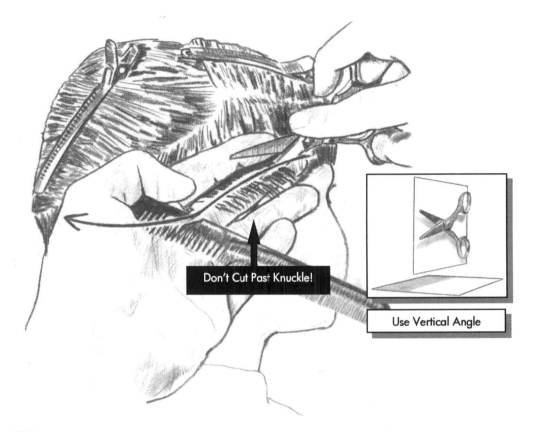

Don't Cut Past Knuckle!

Use Vertical Angle

(Illustration 66): Remember to angle the line slightly downward at this point.

Continue cutting in this manner until your weight-line is completed to the center of the back of the head.

Next, unclip the remaining hair on the right side. Using the same procedure, cut the hair to match.

When the right side is completed, move to the left and repeat the whole procedure.

Blending Bangs with Weight-line

Comb the hair at the left temple area towards the face. Cut on a diagonal line to blend the bangs with the interior weight-line.

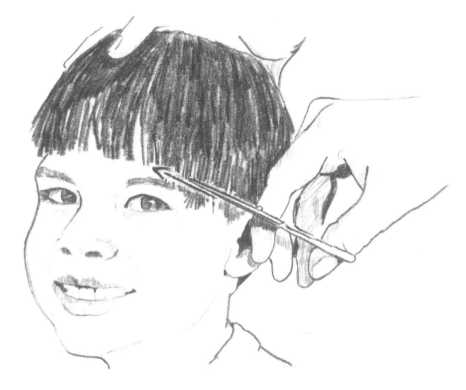

(Illustration 67): Cut on a diagonal line to blend the bangs with the interior weight-line.

NOTE: Please be careful around when cutting around the eye area. A scissor in the eye or cutting off an eyebrow is not good. Not good at all.

Use your free hand to steady the child's head while cutting if necessary. By steady I mean, "Hold on as if your child's vision depended on it"! Repeat on the left side.

Blending the Neck Area

Have your child sit with their head bent slightly forward. The hair should be damp, so re-wet if necessary.

Lightly comb the hair into it's natural growth pattern.

Without holding the hair, cut the neckline against the skin into a softly rounded "U" shape (see Chapter 10, pages 129 - 136).

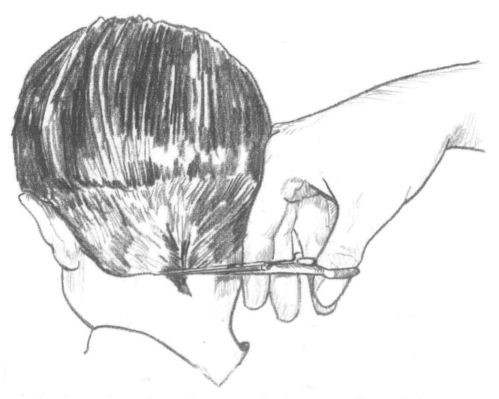

(Illustration 68): Cut the neckline against the skin into a softly rounded "U" shape.

Beginning behind the right ear, comb the hair forward toward the ear and hold as shown.

Make your cut on a line that blends the neckline with the weight-line.

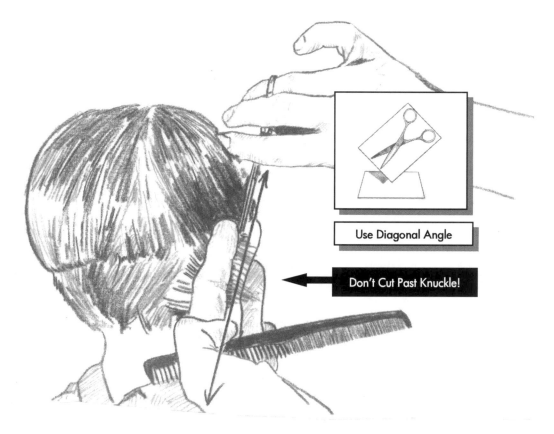

Use Diagonal Angle

Don't Cut Past Knuckle!

(Illustration 69): Cut on a line that blends the neckline with the weight-line.

Now move away from the ear about 1 inch towards the center of the neckline and cut as before. You now have three guides to follow; the neckline, weight-line and previously cut hair from behind the ear.

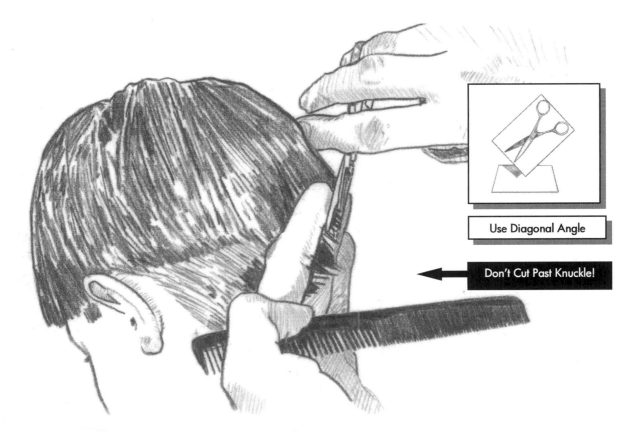

Use Diagonal Angle

Don't Cut Past Knuckle!

(Illustration 70): Now move away from the ear about 1 inch towards the center of the neckline and cut as before.

Continue cutting in this manner until you have reached the center of the neckline.

Move to behind the left ear and repeat this procedure until the neck area is completely blended.

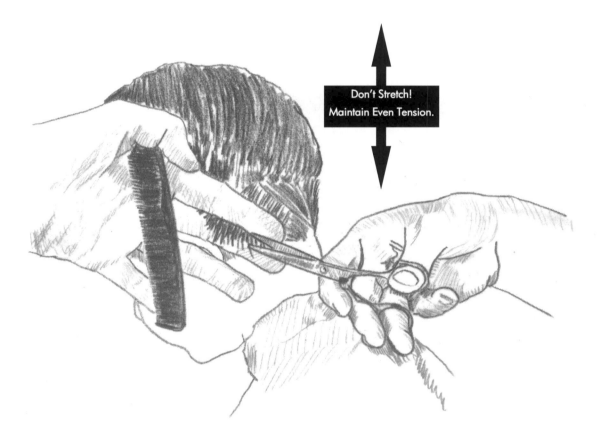

Don't Stretch!
Maintain Even Tension.

(Illustration 71): Move to behind the left ear and repeat this procedure until the neck area is completely blended.

If you desire a fuller, classic wedge as your final result, skip the next section and turn to Chapter 10 (page 119) to learn how to "clean up" and finish your cut.

For a shorter, more layered wedge, continue with the Optional Layered Top.

Optional Layered Top

A classic wedge uses the longer hair on top to contribute to the strong weight-line on the sides.

You may wish to soften this weight-line by creating some layering on top.

To begin, make sure the hair is still damp. Comb child's hair straight back, away from the face.

Create a "Mohawk" section about 1 inch wide along an imaginary line running from the center of the face to the middle of the crown. Comb all other hair down and away from this section.

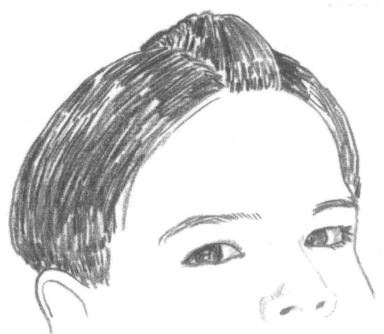

(Illustration 72): Create a "Mohawk" section about 1 inch wide.

Beginning at the portion of this section that is closest to the face, comb hair straight up and grasp between your fingers.

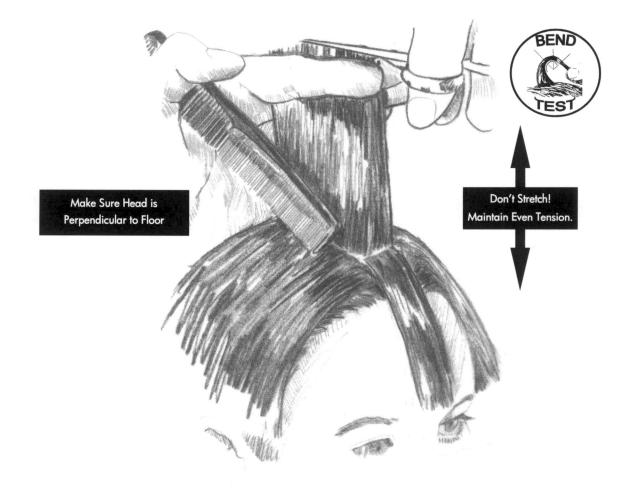

Make Sure Head is
Perpendicular to Floor

BEND
TEST

Don't Stretch!
Maintain Even Tension.

(Illustration 73): Comb hair straight up and grasp between your
fingers.

Using the shorter front lengths as a guide, cut a line from front to back. Make sure that your child's head is upright and straight, and that you are holding the hair in the center of the head along the "Mohawk" line.

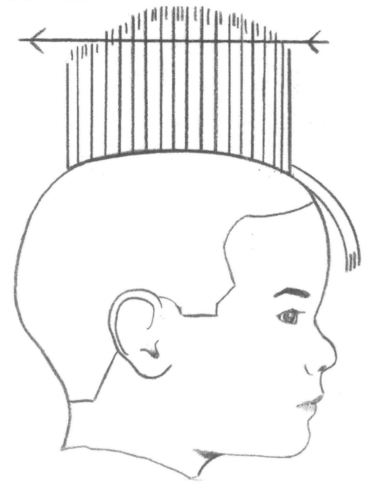

(Illustration 74): Cut a line from front to back.

When the center guide is complete, stand behind your child and comb the guideline hair down into the other hair on the right side of the head.

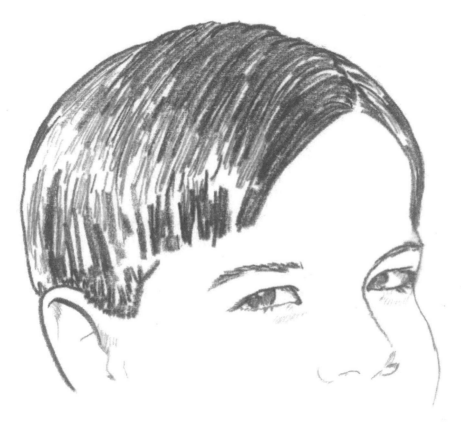

(Illustration 75): Comb the guideline hair down into the other hair on the right side of the head.

Beginning at the front hairline, comb the hair straight up and cut to match your center guideline.

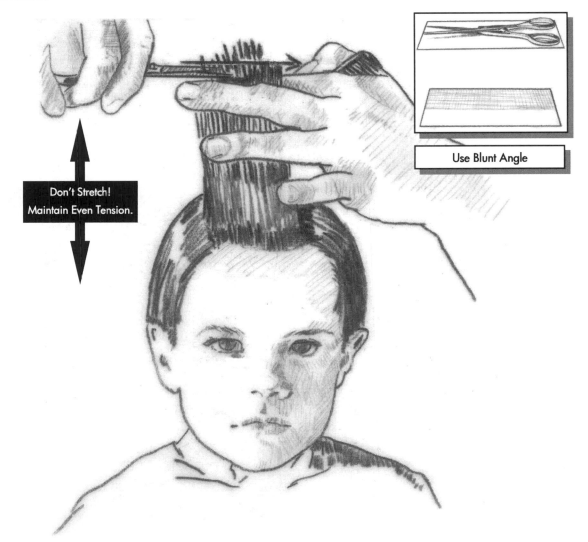

Don't Stretch! Maintain Even Tension.

Use Blunt Angle

(Illustration 76): Comb the hair straight up and cut to match your center guideline.

Now combine hair from the hairline with hair from about 1 inch behind it and cut to match. You now have two guidelines to follow; the center guide and the previously cut hair from the front hairline.

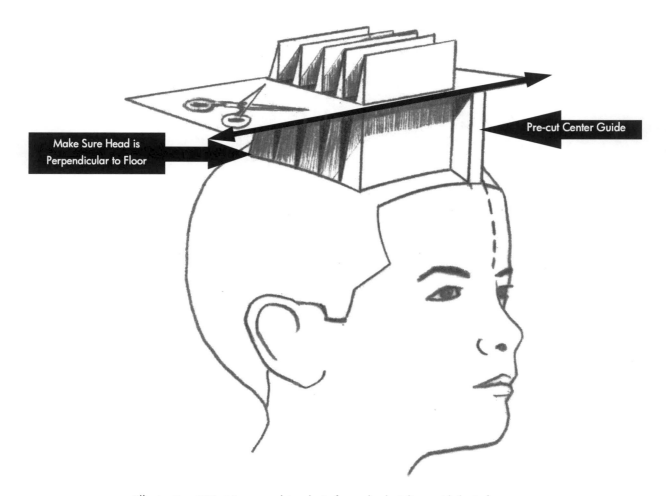

Make Sure Head is Perpendicular to Floor

Pre-cut Center Guide

(Illustration 77): Now combine hair from the hairline with hair from about 1 inch behind it and cut to match. You now have two guidelines to follow; the center guide and the previously cut hair from the front hairline.

Continue cutting in this manner, moving towards the crown in 1-inch wedges until right side is completed

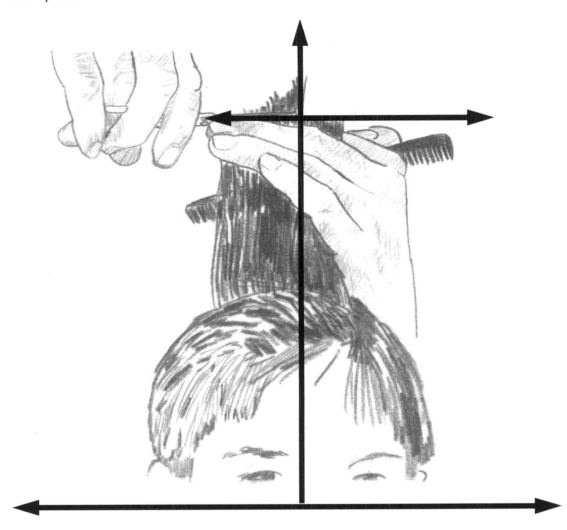

(Illustration 78): Continue cutting in this manner, moving towards the crown in 1-inch wedges until right side is completed

When the right side is finished, comb the hair over to the left side and follow the same procedure.

Once the entire top is layered, turn to Chapter 10 (page 119) to learn how to put the "finishing touches" on your haircut.

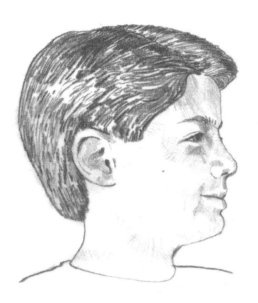

Clippers can be used to create shorter sides and back for this classic boys hairstyle.

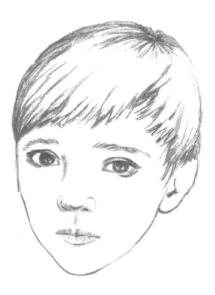

Use thinning shears throughout to achieve the soft edges on this girls short hairstyle. See Chapter 10 (page 119), "Finishing Touches" - "Girls Sideburns" for tips on finishing around the ears.

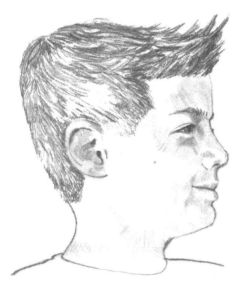

Layer the top with shorter lengths at the crown progressing to longer lengths at the front hairline. Use thinning shears from midway of the hair shaft through the ends to create texture .

The Layered Cut

The layered haircut combines maximum coolness and comfort with an easy-to-care-for, neat appearance that is perfect for active children.

Begin by cutting the bangs according to instructions in Chapter 4 (page 31).

When the bangs are completed, divide the hair into two sections by making a part from just behind one ear across the top of the head to just behind the other ear.

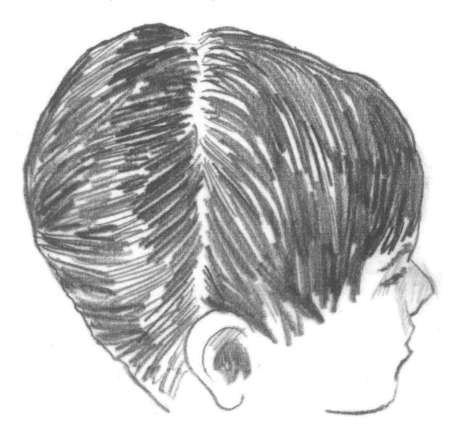

(Illustration 79): When the bangs are completed, divide the hair into two sections.

Next, subdivide hair in the right front section as shown.

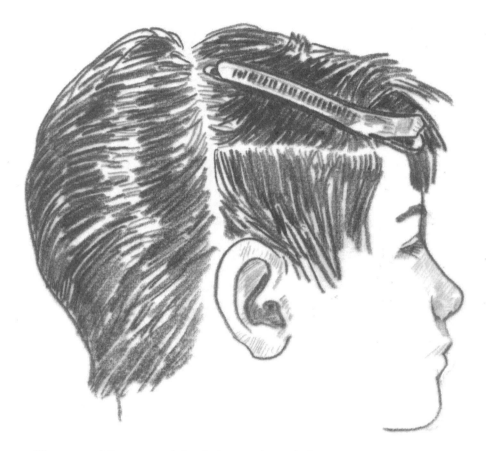

(Illustration 80): Next, subdivide hair in the right front section as shown.

Study the diagram to determine which length will best suit your child.

A. Longest. Cut on a diagonal. This length provides soft, feathery layering that is well suited to girls or boys who like their hair long.

B. Mid Length. A good option for curly hair or to cover protruding ears.

C. Shortest. A neat, comfortable option with a traditional look.

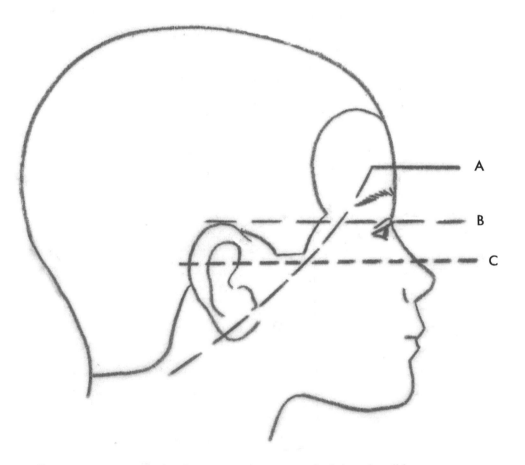

(Illustration 81): Study the diagram to determine which length will best suit your child.

Cutting the Line at the Ear

Begin by combing the hair at the ear up from underneath.

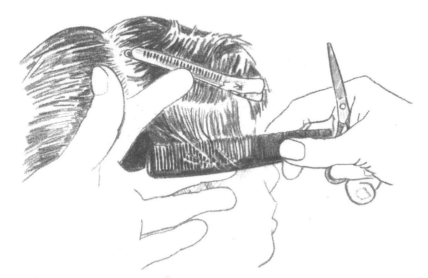

Then comb down from above..

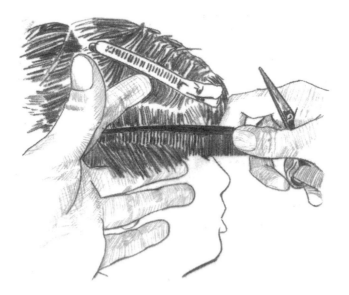

Grasp the hair between your fingers at the level and angle of the desired length.

Now cut to desired length.

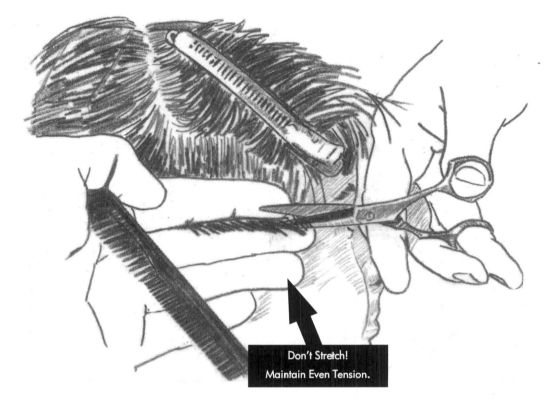

Don't Stretch!
Maintain Even Tension.

(Illustration 84): Grasp the hair between your fingers .

IMPORTANT: Make sure the hand holding the hair is resting firmly against the child's head while you cut this line.

Next, un-clip the remaining hair in the right front section. Using the same procedure, cut to match the previously cut hair.

When the right ear line is completed, move to the left ear and repeat the whole procedure.

Blending Bangs with the Ear Line

Comb the hair at the left temple area towards the face. Cutting against the skin, blend the ear line with the bangs.

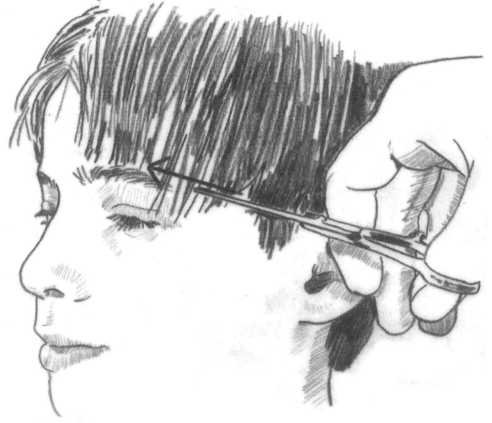

(Illustration 85): Comb the hair at the left temple area towards the face.

Repeat on the right side.

The front "outline" of the haircut is now complete. We will finish all of the layering before cutting the back outline.

NOTE: Please be careful when cutting around the eye area. Eyeballs and scissors are natural enemies. Accidental eyebrow removal is equally undesirable. Watch out for those.

Layering the Top

To begin, comb your child's hair straight back off the face.

Create a "Mohawk" section about 1 inch wide along an imaginary line running from the center of the face to the middle of the crown.

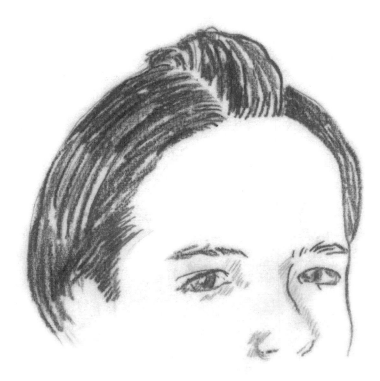

(Illustration 86): Create a "Mohawk" section.

Comb the rest of the hair down and away from this section.

Starting at the portion of this section that is closest to the face, comb the hair straight up and grasp it between your fingers.

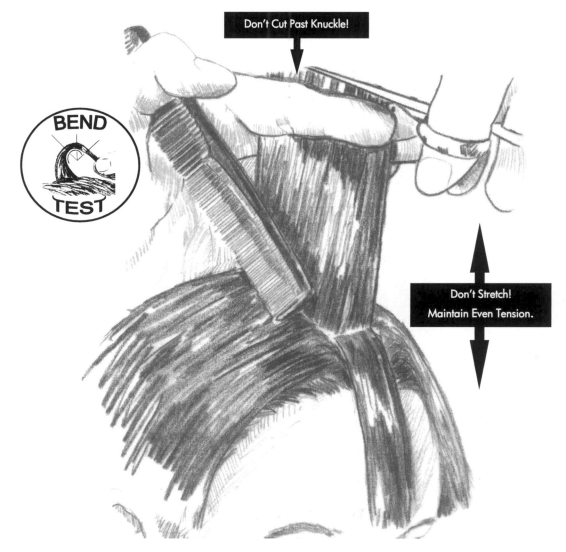

(Illustration 87): Start at the portion of this section that is closest to the face.

Allow some of the bang hair to fall back onto the forehead as a precaution against cutting into the established bang line.

Using the shorter front lengths as a guide, cut a line from front to back as shown. Make sure that your child's head is upright and straight, and that you are holding the hair in the center of the head along the "Mohawk" line.

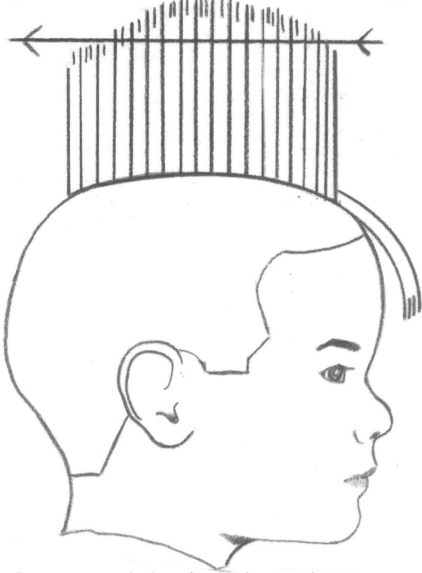

(Illustration 88): Use the shorter front lengths as a guide.

When the center guide is complete, stand behind your child and comb the guideline hair down into the other hair on the right side of the head.

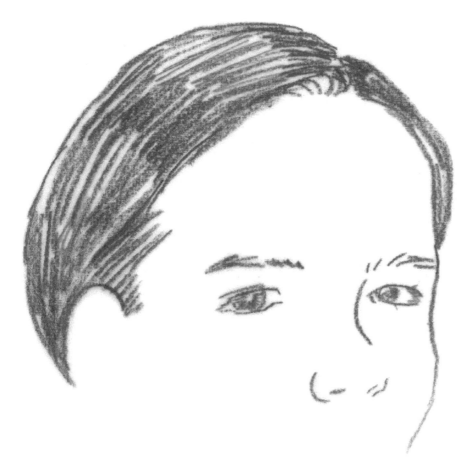

(Illustration 89): Stand behind your child and comb the guideline hair down into the other hair on the right side of the head.

Beginning at the front hairline, comb the hair straight up and cut to match your center guideline.

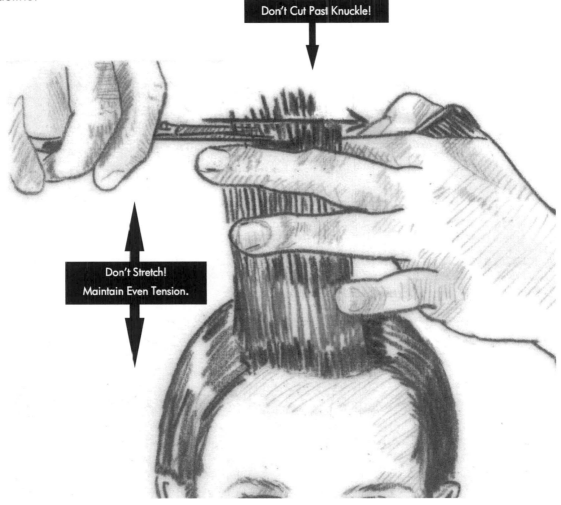

(Illustration 90): Comb the hair straight up and cut to match your center guideline.

Now combine hair from the hairline with hair from about 1 inch behind it and cut to match. You now have two guidelines to follow: the center guideline and the previously cut hair from the front hairline.

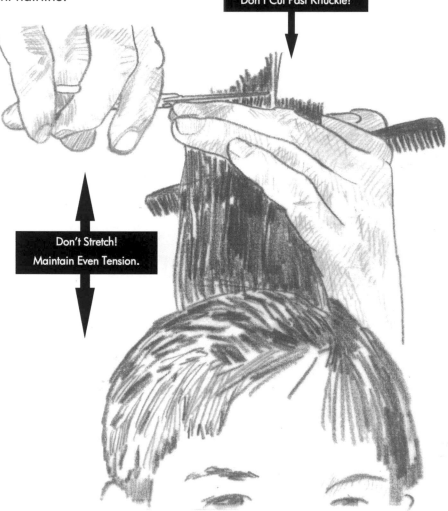

Don't Cut Past Knuckle!

Don't Stretch!
Maintain Even Tension.

(Illustration 91): Combine hair from the hairline with hair from about 1 inch behind it and cut to match.

Continue cutting in this manner, moving toward the crown in 1-inch wedges until the right top is completed.

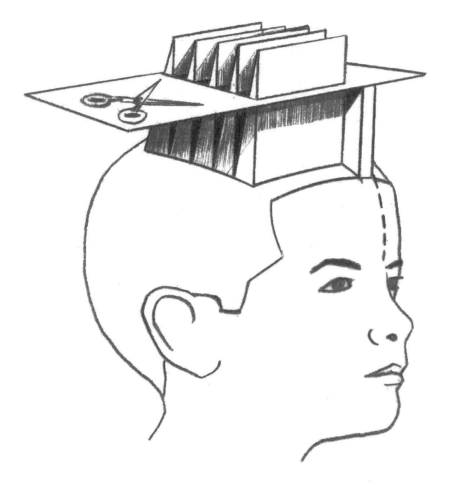

(Illustration 92): Continue cutting in this manner, moving toward the crown in 1-inch wedges until the right top is completed.

When the right top is finished, comb the hair over to the left and follow the same procedure.

Layering the Sides and Back

Once the entire top is layered, prepare to layer the right side of the head by combing the top hair over to the right.

While standing behind your child, part off a 1-inch wide vertical section at the right front hairline and hold between your fingers.

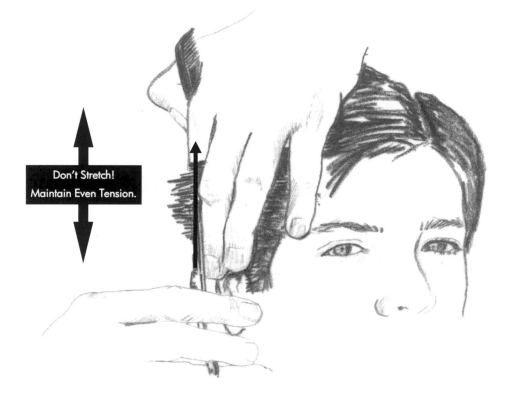

Don't Stretch!
Maintain Even Tension.

(Illustration 93): Part off a 1-inch wide vertical section at the right front hairline and hold between your fingers.

You have two guides to go by; the previously cut hair from the top (A) and the previously cut hair at the ear (B).

Make a straight cut to connect these two points.

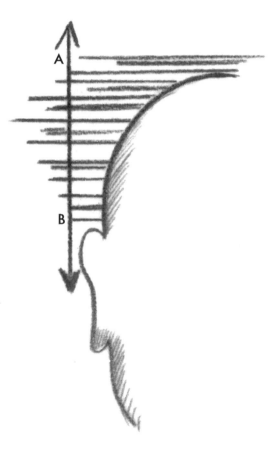

(Illustration 94): Make a straight cut to connect these two points.

Now combine the previously cut hair from the right front hairline with the uncut hair about 1 inch back and cut to match. This is the same method you used to layer the top, only it's done sideways.

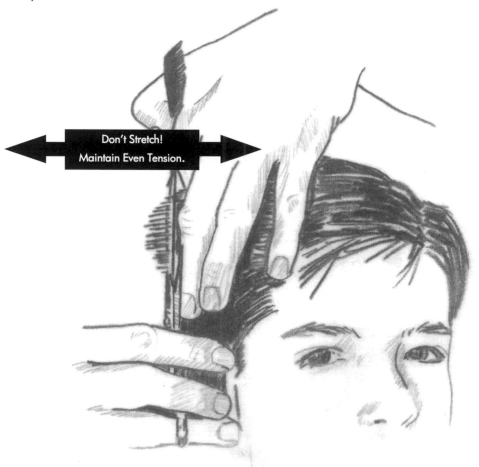

Don't Stretch!
Maintain Even Tension.

(Illustration 95): Combine the previously cut hair from the right front hairline with the uncut.

Continue in this manner until you reach the center of the back of the head.

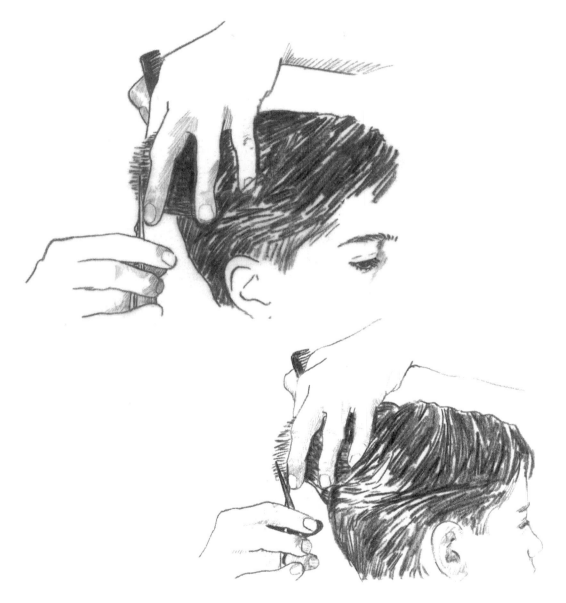

(Illustration 96): Continue until you reach the center of the back of the head.

Next, grasp the hair behind the ear as shown. Cut the hair in a straight, vertical line to match the previously cut hair in the area above the ear.

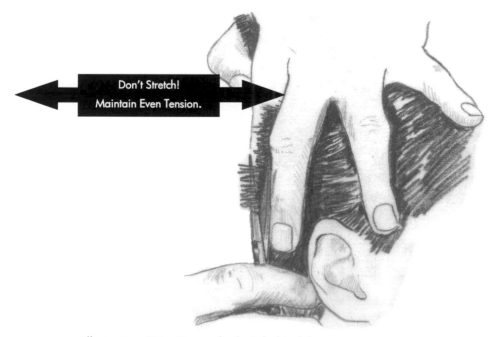

Don't Stretch!
Maintain Even Tension.

(Illustration 97): Grasp the hair behind the ear.

Now combine the previously cut hair from behind the ear with the uncut hair about 1 inch back and cut to match.

Continue cutting in this manner, moving toward the center of the back of the head in 1-inch wedges until the right side is completely layered.

When the right side is finished, comb the top hair over to the left side and follow the same procedure.

Once you have layered the entire head, turn to Chapter 10 to learn how to put the "finishing touches" on your haircut.

For more information on children's haircutting, videos and deals on haircutting tools visit
www.HowToCutChildrensHair.com

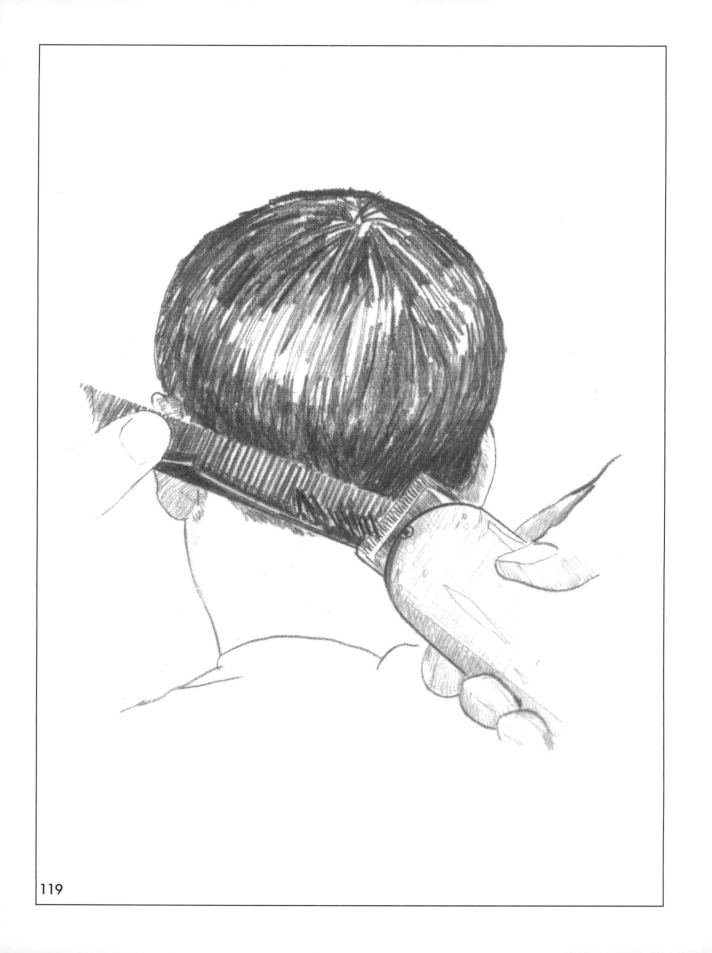

Finishing Touches

Once the general shaping has been completed, short haircuts may require a few special "finishing touches". These steps should be saved until after the length and bulk have been removed so that the direction of growth in the hairline can be clearly seen.

How you shape the neckline and ear areas are slightly different for boys and girls. As a general rule, boys' short haircuts are finished with squared sideburns and wide, squared-off necklines. Often boys' short haircuts will be very close-cut or tapered in the sideburns, ear and neckline areas.

In contrast, girls' short haircuts usually have soft, fringed sideburns with more length and fullness at the ear than boys. Girls' short necklines, whether tapered or fringed, usually have a more narrow, rounded or pointed shape.

These are general guidelines, not rules. Current fashion, comfort and a child's individual characteristics should determine the final choices.

Ear Area

In very short haircuts you may want the hair cut so that it does not touch the ear.

Simply fold the top of the ear downward. This doesn't hurt despite the face your child may make. With your free hand, comb the hair around the ear downward and towards the face.

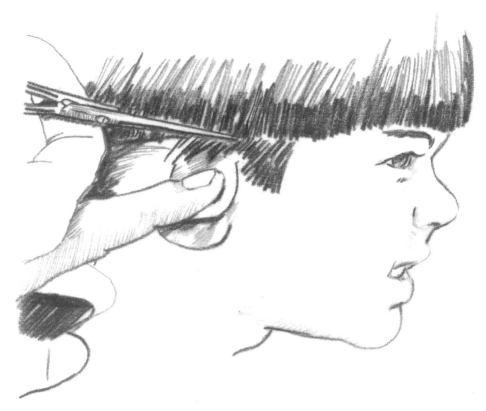

(Illustration 98): Fold the top of the ear downward.

Using scissors or electric clippers, begin cutting behind the ear. Follow the natural contour of the hairline, stopping in the front of the ear where the ear attaches to the head.

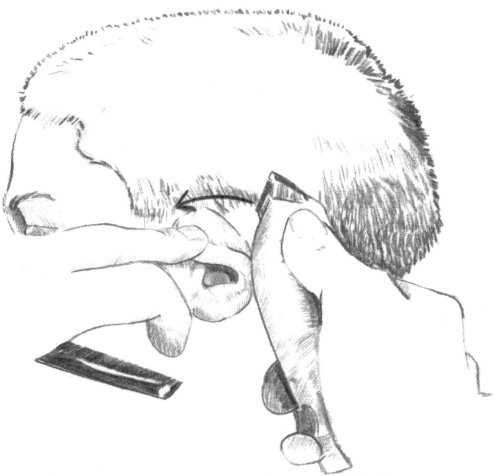

(Illustration 99): Use scissors or electric clippers to cut behind the ear.

Boys Sideburns

Once the area around the ear is finished, use your comb to direct the sideburn hair towards the ear.

Use scissors or clippers to cut off any hair that touches the ear.

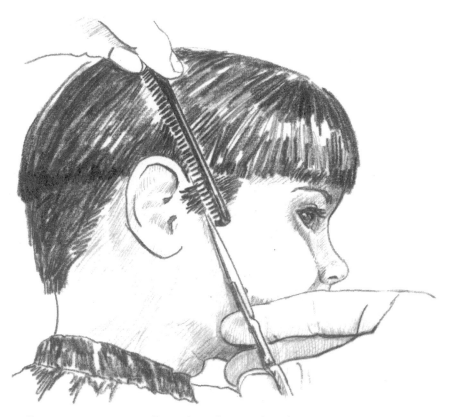

(Illustration 100): Cut off any hair that touches the ear.

Now comb the sideburn straight down and square off the bottom by cutting a line that is parallel to the floor. The standard length for boys' sideburns is level with the top of the cheekbone.

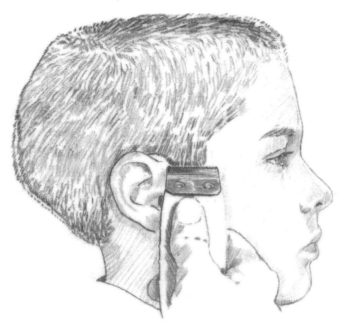

If the sideburn seems too thick, lift up the hair with your comb and trim off some of the bulk. you may vary the length to adapt to your child's face.

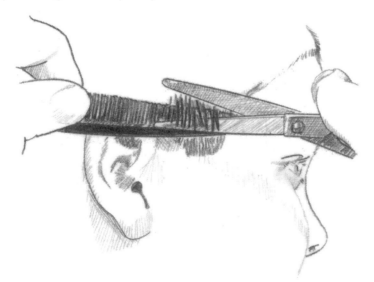

Girls' Sideburns

Generally, girls' sideburns can be left a little longer and softer edged than boys. Cut with the tips of your scissors to create a softer look. Leaving a little extra length in this area will help prevent others from mistaking your short-haired girl for a short-haired boy!

Begin by combing the sideburn hair towards the ear. Snip off any hair that touches the ear.

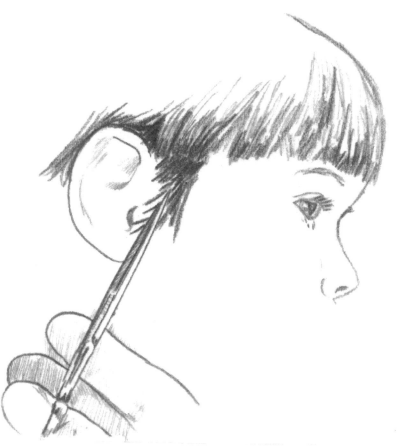

(Illustration 103): Begin by combing the sideburn hair towards the ear.
Snip off any hair that touches the ear.

Next, comb the sideburn towards the face. Snip off any hair that extends onto the cheek or into the eye area.

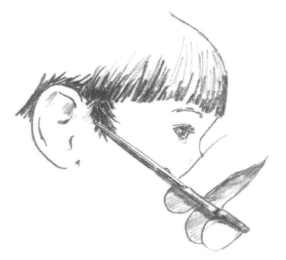

Now comb the hair downward. Use your scissor tips to snip off excessive length and bulk to create a soft, feathery effect.

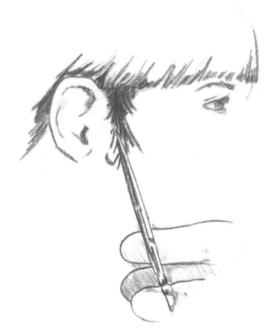

Necklines

Due to a wide variety of possible growth patterns and textures, the neckline can sometimes be the most perplexing area to cut.

These same variables, when approached creatively, can become a distinctive part of your child's appearance.

Save this area of the haircut until after any layering or bulk removal has been completed. This allows you to see the natural growth patterns more easily.

General Suggestions

- Have your child sit with their back facing a mirror. Looking at the reversed image in the mirror will help you spot any imbalance in the shape.

- <u>Always</u> comb the hair following the natural growth direction. No amount of combing will ever make an upward-growing hairline lie down.

- <u>Always</u> cut against the skin with no tension or stretch on the hair.

- Boys' necklines are usually short and somewhat wide and square. Girls' necklines are usually narrower than boys with a softer edge. Use the scissor tips to cut the outline on girls' necklines.

- Cut the base of the neckline first, then cut behind the ears.

Always cut against the skin with no tension or stretch on the hair.

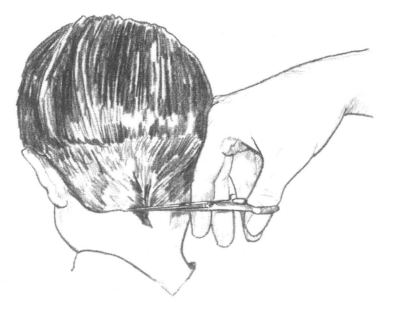

Cut the base of the neckline first, then cut behind the ears.

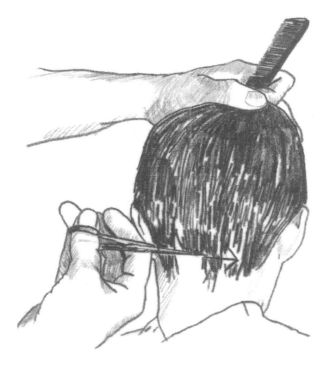

Five Typical Neckline Growth Patterns and How to Cut Them

Look through the following examples and find the illustration that most closely resembles your child's neckline.

Cut the neckline into the corresponding suggested shape, making sure that the child's head is in a normal, upright position. Bending the head forward causes the skin to stretch, which causes the hairline to move and distort from it's normal shape.

All of these shapes should be cut with the hair against the skin and with as little stretching as you can manage.

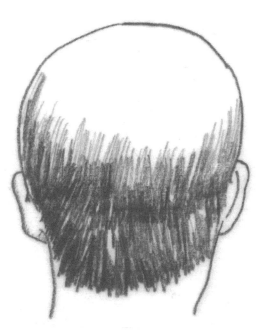

(Illustration 108): <u>Symmetrical Growth Pattern</u>:
Smooth, evenly distributed downward growth.

Suggested Shapes for Symmetrical Growth Pattern

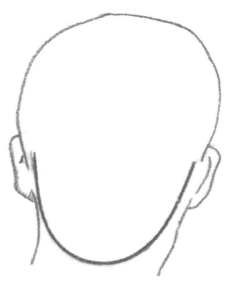

(Illustration 109): "U" Shape Neckline

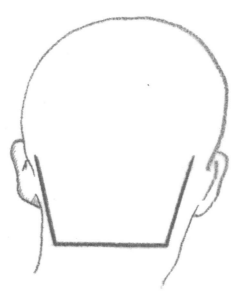

(Illustration 110): Squared Neckline

Chapter 10 / Finishing Touches

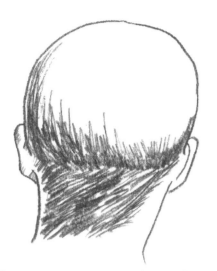

(Illustration 111): <u>Diagonal Growth Pattern</u>:
All hair grows from one side on a downward angle towards the other side.

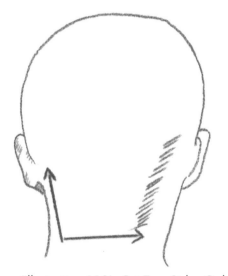

(Illustration 112): <u>Cut Two Sides Only</u>:
The side that the Growth pattern originates from will create it's own line.
Cut against the growth direction at the base.

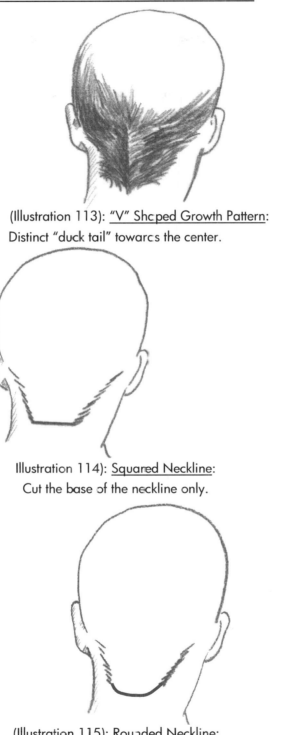

(Illustration 113): "V" Shaped Growth Pattern:
Distinct "duck tail" towards the center.

Illustration 114): Squared Neckline:
Cut the base of the neckline only.

(Illustration 115): Rounded Neckline:
Cut the base of the neckline only.

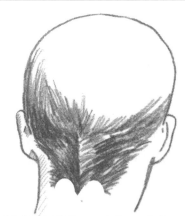

(Illustration 116): <u>"M" Shaped Growth Pattern</u>:

The hair at the base of the neckline grows upward, then down towards the center.

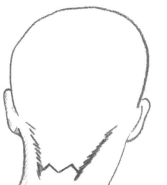

(Illustration 117): <u>Natural Neckline</u> :

Simply neaten and reinforce the "M" for a distinctive look.

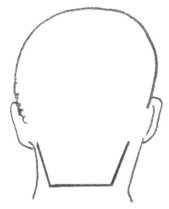

(Illustration 118): <u>Squared Neckline</u>:

Cut into the hair at the base of the neckline to create a straight line.

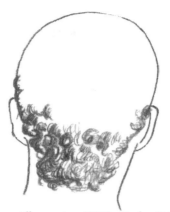

(Illustration 119): <u>Curly, Wavy Growth Pattern</u>:
The more curl there is, the more readily the neckline will hold a shape.

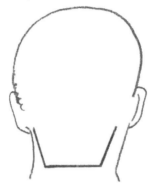

(Illustration 120): <u>Squared Neckline</u> :
Cut against the skin *without holding the hair* in any way.

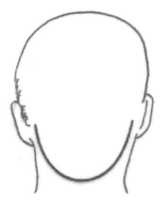

(Illustration 121): <u>Rounded Neckline</u>:
Cut against the skin *without holding the hair* in any way.

If you feel that further bulk needs to be removed in the neckline area, lift the hair with your comb and use scissors or clippers to create a more closely fitted shape.

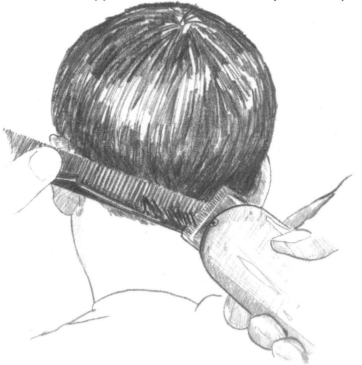

(Illustration 122): Use scissors or clippers to create a more closely fitted shape.

Shaving the Neck Area

The final step in any short haircut is to remove any excess hair on the neck. Electric clippers will do the job nicely. However, a safety razor with a little soapy water applied first will give you the smoothest results. Be sure to shave with the direction of the hair growth to prevent ingrown hairs. PLEASE USE EXTREME CAUTION. If you are not confident about your shaving skills, don't do it. Just snip it as short as you can with the tips of the scissors.

Creating Texture

Texture is the effect of removing the blunt edges of a haircut with thinning shears or by <u>carefully</u> using the points of the scissors to snip small pieces. Thinning shears are the best tool for beginners to use. Texturizing is an advanced technique and I recommend that novices use it sparingly or not at all.

Wait until all of the main steps of the haircut are finished and the hair is dry and styled. Then begin inserting the thinning shears into the are you want more texture in and make a sample cut. Comb out the loose, cut hairs and observe the effect of that one stroke.. (see illustration 123 below)

Now continue this process in any areas that need more texturizing until the haircut looks the way you want it to look. This is a visual, creative process and there are no definite rule about how much or how little hair to remove.

If you are trying to create a spiky effect on the top of a layered haircut, be sure to do the "Bend Test" and make sure you are not thinning any closer to the scalp than the first bend.

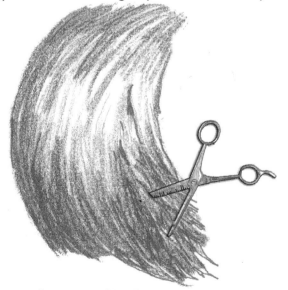

(Illustration 123): Creating texture.

Notes

For more information on children's haircutting, videos and deals on haircutting tools visit
www.HowToCutChildrensHair.com

137